Endometriosis

Advances in Reproductive Endocrinology

VOLUME 1

Endometriosis

Edited by RW Shaw

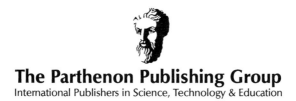

The Parthenon Publishing Group
International Publishers in Science, Technology & Education

Casterton Hall, Carnforth,
Lancs, LA6 2LA, UK

120 Mill Road, Park Ridge,
New Jersey, USA

Published in the UK by
The Parthenon Publishing Group Limited
Casterton Hall, Carnforth,
Lancs, LA6 2LA, England

Published in the USA by
The Parthenon Publishing Group Inc.
120 Mill Road,
Park Ridge,
New Jersey 07656, USA

British Library Catologuing-in-Publication Data
Endometriosis.
  1. Women.   Endometriosis
  I. Shaw, Robert W. (Robert Wayne)   II. Series
  618.14

  ISBN 1-85070-297-7
  ISBN 0-929858-48-4 U.S.

Library of Congress Cataloging-in-Publication Data
International Workshops in Reproductive Endocrinology (1989 :
  Cambridge, England)
    Endometriosis / International Workshops in Reproductive
  Endocrinology ; edited by R.W. Shaw.
        p.   cm.
    Based on the workshops held in Cambridge, England, Sept. 1989.
    Includes bibliographical references.
    ISBN 0-929858-48-4 : $55.00
    1. Endometriosis - - Congresses.   I. Shaw, Robert W. (Robert Wayne)
  II. Title.
    [DNLM: 1. Endometriosis - - congresses.   WP 390 I617e 1989]
  RG483.E53I58   1989
  618.1'42 - - dc20
  DNLM/DLC
  for Library of Congress   90-6921
                                                                    CIP

First published 1990

Composition by Ryburn Typesetting Ltd, Halifax, England
Printed and bound in Great Britain by
Butler and Tanner, Frome and London

Contents

List of principal contributors

D.H. Barlow
Nuffield Department of Obstetrics
    and Gynaecology
John Radcliffe Maternity Hospital
Oxford
UK

A. Bergqvist
Department of Obstetrics and
    Gynaecology
Malmö General Hospital
S-214 0l Malmö
Sweden

G.B. Candiani
Ia Clinica Ostetrica e Ginecologica
Via Commenda 12
20122 Milano
Italy

J. Donnez
Department of Gynaecology
Catholic University of Leuven
Cliniques Universitaires St. Luc
Avenue Hippocrate 10
B-1200 Brussels
Belgium

M. Dowsett
Department of Biochemical
    Endocrinology
Royal Marsden Hospital
Fulham Road
London SW3 6JJ
UK

J.L.H. Evers
Department of Obstetrics and
    Gynaecology
Academisch Ziekenhuis Maastricht,
P.O. Box 1918
6201 BX Maastricht
Holland

B.J.A. Furr
Bioscience 1
ICI Pharmaceuticals,
Mereside
Alderley Park
Macclesfield
Cheshire SK10 4TG
UK

A.F. Henderson
Menopause Clinic
Dulwich Hospital
East Dulwich Grove
London SE22
UK

P.R. Koninckx
Department of Obstetrics and
  Gynaecology
University Hospital
Gasthuisberg
Catholic University of Leuven
B-3000 Leuven
Belgium

L.R. Malinak
Center for Reproductive Medicine
  and Surgery
Baylor College of Medicine
6550 Fannin # 801
Houston
Texas 77030
USA

K.-W. Schweppe
Department of Obstetrics and
  Gynaecology
Academic Teaching Hospital of the
  University of Göttingen
Lange Strasse 38
D-2910 Westerstede
Federal Republic of Germany

R.W. Shaw
Academic Department of Obstetrics
  and Gynaecology
Royal Free Hospital School of
  Medicine
Pond Street
London NW3 2QG
UK

C. Sutton
St. Luke's Hospital
Warren Road
Guilford
Surrey GU1 3NT
UK

E.J. Thomas
Department of Obstetrics and
  Gynaecology
Newcastle General Hospital
Westgate Road
Newcastle-upon-Tyne
UK

P.L. Venturini
Clinica Ostetrica e Ginecologica
University of Genoa
Viale Benedetto XV
16132 Genoa
Italy

J.M. Wheeler
Center for Reproductive Medicine
  and Surgery
Baylor College of Medicine
6550 Fannin # 801
Houston
Texas 77030
USA

Foreword

Endometriosis is one of the commonest benign gynaecological conditions, yet although it is so widespread, there is much which is poorly understood with regard to its aetiology and pathogenesis. The condition has aroused much interest and controversy in recent years with regard to its diagnosis, infertility association and treatment. The time is thus right to review all of the above aspects and to assess newer medical and surgical treatment approaches.

In September 1989, under the kind sponsorship of ICI Pharmaceuticals, the first in a series of International Workshops in Reproductive Endocrinology was held. A group of international specialists from nine countries met and discussed the topic of endometriosis. Aspects reviewed were its clinical presentation, diagnosis, pathogenesis, pathophysiology, deep infiltration and recurrence. Current medical therapies were critically evaluated as was the association of endometriosis with infertility. In addition, the newer treatment approach utilising GnRH analogues and that using laser surgical procedures were compared with the role of hormone replacement therapy (HRT) when radical surgery is finally performed.

In all, a comprehensive evaluation of this enigmatic disease took place which should provide clinicians with an up-to-date review of past, present and future thoughts surrounding the aetiology, pathogenesis and management of endometriosis.

Professor Robert W. Shaw
Academic Department of Obstetrics and Gynaecology
Royal Free Hospital School of Medicine
London

1

Endometriosis: clinical presentation and diagnosis

D.H. Barlow and S.H. Kennedy

INTRODUCTION

Endometriosis is a possible diagnosis in a large range of clinical presentations in women from the menarche to the menopause[1], and even beyond the menopause[2]. Since the diagnosis can generally only be made by surgical intervention and since some women with endometriosis are asymptomatic we can only guess at the true incidence in the female population. Recently Wheeler[3] has indicated that endometriosis might be present in as many as 10% of the female population of reproductive age, based on surgical findings in women undergoing surgery where endometriosis was not a likely diagnosis. Pauerstein[4] has reviewed the literature on the prevalence of endometriosis, and he clearly demonstrates that the reason for the diagnostic intervention influences the detected prevalence (Table 1).

SYMPTOMATOLOGY

The localization of the disease process largely determines the symptoms a woman may experience. Many years ago Scott and Te Linde[5] presented the sites of endometriosis detected in a series of 516 cases. They showed the ovaries to be the commonest site followed by pelvic peritoneal

Table 1   Prevalence of the reported diagnosis of endometriosis in different clinical situations

Situation	Number of studies	Total number of cases		Range
Gynaecological laparotomy	9	432/33 598	(0.1%)	0.1–9%
Pelvic pain laparoscopy	8	180/960	(18.8%)	4.5–32%
Infertile laparoscopy	5	140/989	(14.2%)	4.5–33%

(adapted from Pauerstein[4])

surfaces and the posterior aspect of the uterus. Each of the other possible sites involved only a handful of cases. In an infertility population of 182 women, Jenkins and colleagues[6] similarly noted the ovary to be a major site (54.9%) followed by the posterior broad ligament (35.2%), the anterior or posterior pouch of Douglas (each 34%) and the uterosacral ligaments (28%). Since endometriosis is outstandingly a pelvic disease with extra-pelvic involvement being relatively uncommon, it is appropriate to limit discussion mainly to pelvic disease in this account of clinical presentation and diagnosis.

The classic symptom of endometriosis is pelvic pain associated with menstruation or the immediate premenstrual phase. The basis for the pain is uncertain but could reflect stretching of tissues by the menstrual process, an effect of the local production of prostaglandins by the endometriotic implants or it might relate to tissue damage and adhesion formation. It is clear that there is a huge variation in the extent of symptomatic distress and that this does not correlate with the extent of observed disease. Many women found to have endometriosis are asymptomatic and some of them have severe disease discovered after the incidental detection of an ovarian mass or during infertility laparoscopy. In some asymptomatic women it may be that the disease has disrupted pelvic sensation.

Another classic symptom of endometriosis is deep dyspareunia probably resulting from the stretching of affected pelvic tissues such as a fixed retroverted uterus or pressure on diseased ovaries, uterosacral ligaments or rectovaginal septum. It should be noted that dyspareunia caused by lesions in these areas is a variable finding. In the Brisbane series of 717 women only one in four of those sexually active and with pouch of Douglas involvement admitted to dyspareunia[7].

There may be a link between menstrual history and the occurence of endometriosis, but this may relate more to certain menstrual patterns such as short cycles or heavy loss favouring the development of endometriosis rather than being a consequence of the disease.

Infertility is a problem for some women who are found to have endometriosis and many of them are otherwise asymptomatic. It is still unclear to what extent endometriosis causes infertility; a topic to be considered by another presentation at this meeting. Other symptoms are less common and include cyclical rectal bleeding and haematuria if the relevant tracts are involved.

PHYSICAL EXAMINATION

Some aspects of clinical examination may raise the level of suspicion that pelvic endometriosis might be present. These include finding an ovarian mass or masses, thickening or tenderness in the uterosacral or pouch of Douglas areas and fixed uterine retroversion. However, the diagnosis generally has to rest on direct vizualization of lesions, usually by laparoscopy.

LAPAROSCOPIC DIAGNOSIS

Laparoscopy permits a detailed exploration of the pelvic environment and the detection of endometriotic deposits not possible by other means, including laparotomy. The extent to which classic blackish powder-burn lesions must be confirmed histologically remains a matter of opinion but it is clear that attempted pathological confirmation fails in some cases. Portuando[8] reported a 70% confirmation rate using light microscopy whereas Vasquez and colleagues and Murphy and colleagues[9,10] reported confirmation rates of approximately 85% using light and electron microscopic methods.

There is now good evidence that peritoneal black or blue-black lesions perhaps with associated fibrosis or adhesions represent only part of the spectrum of visual manifestations of peritoneal endometriosis which may be demonstrated by biopsy. Redwine[11] has emphasized that most peritoneal endometriosis is not black and that many small haemorrhagic and non-haemorrhagic lesions represent what may be stages in the progression of the disease. Jansen and Russell[12] have correlated these less classic appearances with the rate of biopsy confirmation indicating good rates of confirmation for white opacified peritoneum (81%), red flame-like lesions (81%), glandular lesions visually resembling endometrium (67%) and reasonable correlations for subovarian adhesions (50%), yellow-brown patches (47%) and circular peritoneal defects (45%). The problem of diagnosis has been further compounded by the evidence that some visually normal peritoneum can be shown to contain endometriosis on pathological examination[10,13]. The importance of detecting the more subtle appearance is emphasized by the *in vitro* studies of Vernon[14] and colleagues who measured endometriotic implant production of prostaglandin F (PGF) which is one possible mediator of the effect of the disease on fertility. They found the highest production to be from reddish petechial lesions with less from brown and least from black lesions. On the basis of these studies it is clear that careful laparoscopy by an experienced surgeon is essential if cases are not to be missed and where there is any doubt there is a need for biopsy confirmation. It is possible that this diagnostic difficulty is the basis for the confusion in the literature on the effects of endometriosis on the intraperitoneal environment.

NON-INVASIVE DIAGNOSTIC TECHNIQUES

It is unsatisfactory that an invasive surgical procedure must be performed in order to diagnose or assess the progress of endometriosis or its treatment. Attemps to provide a non-invasive test which might have a high sensitivity and specificity for endometriosis have so far eluded investigators. It would be valuable even if we had a technique which might either exclude endometriosis or raise the level of clinical suspicion sufficiently to improve the selection of those who need to undergo laparoscopy. This could be of particular importance if the resources of laparoscopy were under pressure. Currently the avenues explored have involved serum markers or the use of imaging techniques.

Serum markers

The most widely tested serum marker for endometriosis has been the use of the monoclonal antibody OC-125 which was raised by injecting mice with a human ovarian cancer cell line[15]. The antigen expressed by the tumour was designated CA-125 and is a high molecular weight (>200 000) glycoprotein. This antigen has now been shown to be expressed by many tissues present in the pelvis as well as more distant sites including pericardium and pleura. Grossly elevated levels have been useful as a marker for ovarian cancer but moderate elevation has been observed in endometriosis, particularly in severe disease[16,17]. In these studies of serum levels, the sensitivity and specificity (at >35 U/ml cut off) have proved inadequate for its use as a screening test for endometriosis. Recently Pittaway and Douglas[18] have used a lower upper limit at >16 U/ml in 163 women with pelvic pain. They reported an overall sensitivity of 80% and specificity of 94% (Table 2). In our own smaller series of 28 endometriosis patients even the >16 U/ml cut off failed to detect 43% of AFS severe cases[19]. Levels of CA-125 in peritoneal fluid have been examined as a means of improving detection of endometriosis, but although levels are higher in peritoneal fluid than serum there are no clear differences between endometriosis and controls[20,21].

An alternative approach which is now being explored is the detection

Table 2 The use of serum CA-125 in the prediction of endometriosis in women with pelvic pain

Diagnosis	n	*CA-125* *>16 U/ml*	
No endometriosis	81	5	(6%)
pelvic inflam.	28	3	(11%)
Endometriosis	82	66	(80%)
minimal	25	13	(52%)
mild	29	25	(86%)
moderate	19	19	(100%)
severe	9	9	(100%)

(from Pittaway and Douglas[18])

of circulating antibodies directed against endometrium in women with endometriosis. There is evidence that women with endometriosis may exhibit abnormal levels of autoantibodies including antinuclear factor and lupus anticoagulant[22]. It has been possible for some time to detect organ specific autoantibodies directed against endometrium using a variety of methods[23-25]. Chihal and colleagues suggested that an anti-endometrial antibody assay might be used as a test for endometriosis[25]. They employed a passive haemagglutination assay and reported a 70% sensitivity and 100% specificity. The measurement of antibodies directed against endometrium has been complicated by a relatively high level of endogenous immunoglobulin in that tissue. In order to overcome this problem we have explored a double antibody indirect immunohistochemical technique in which the thin sections of endometrium are first incubated with an enzyme-linked antiglobulin which reacts to give a brown colour on exposure to substrate and indicates the endogenous immunoglobulin. The tissue is then incubated with the serum to be tested, then a second enzyme-linked antiglobulin conjugated with alkaline phosphatase which develops to a pink colour. Using this qualitative double antibody technique we have detected binding in the sera of 14 out of 40 women with endometriosis (35%) compared with 1 of 40 controls (2.5%)[26]. Since a quantitative assay system is to be preferred for the development of a diagnostic test we have subsequently developed an enzyme-linked immunoabsorbant assay (ELISA) for anti-endometrial antibodies based on the use of human endometrium. ELISA methods make possible a rapid, sensitive and quantitative antibody assessment. Data on an ELISA based on bovine endometrium has very recently been presented by Moncayo and Moncayo–Naveda[27]. They report the detection of anti-endometrial antibodies in 64% of 14 endometriosis cases. We have used proliferative human endometrium and from this prepared a gland extract used to coat ELISA plates. The test sera are applied to the plates and the binding of anti-endometrial antibodies from the sera is detected by an enzymatic colourometric reaction. Preliminary results have revealed significantly higher antibody levels in sera from 35 women with endometriosis before medical treatment than after 6 months treatment[28]. The pre-treatment anti-endometrial antibody level was significantly higher than in female controls and in male and umbilical cord control sera. Further work is needed before we can discover if such quantitative assays can have a place in the detection or monitoring of endometriosis.

Imaging techniques

We now have a wide range of imaging techiques which can be used to examine the pelvis but in general their value in endometriosis has been limited. Pelvic ultrasound will demonstrate ovarian cystic masses but will not reliably differentiate these from other cysts and will not detect peritoneal disease. In a comparison of a pre-laparoscopy ultrasound with operative findings Friedman and colleagues observed very poor correlation with an accurate scan prediction in only four of 37 cases[29]. Computerized tomography (CT) offers better definition than ultrasound in many situations but has not established a role in the assessment of pelvic endometriosis. An unusual case where CT was of some value was in the assessment of a suspected recurrence of an abdominal wall scar endometrioma where the CT image helped in the monitoring of initial medical treatment and then in the planning of surgery[30]. Another expensive imaging technique whose role in gynaecology is still emerging is Magnetic Resonance Imaging (MRI). There have been a few reports on the application of MRI to adnexal masses, and it is suggested that endometriotic material might be detected via its higher blood content[31,32], but Butler and colleagues[33] have reported a significant overlap between endometriomas and cystadenomas on MRI. These scanning methods have little to offer in the detection of peritoneal disease whereas our preliminary evidence suggests that it may be possible to use immunoscintigraphic imaging to detect peritoneal disease.

Since it was clear that endometriotic tissue was expressing CA-125 which could be detected in the circulation after shedding, we explored whether the antigen could be detected at the site of expression by applying immunoscintigraphic methods. This involved injecting labelled OC-125 F(ab')$_2$ fragments then using a gamma camera to detect the sites of binding. The preliminary study involved ^{131}I as label and it was possible to demonstrate binding[34]. The lower radiation dose [111]I which permitted finer focussing was then obtained and we screened, pre-laparoscopy, 21 women complaining of pain or infertility. We detected pelvic uptake in 16 women many of whom had endometriosis but some had adhesions of uncertain origin. There were cases with minimal endometriosis who gave no detectable pelvic uptake. If considered as a screening method to determine the likelihood of finding pelvic pathology the sensitivity was 91% and the specificity 60%.

We have seen that there are promising areas of investigation being currently pursued into the non-invasive highlighting of women who might have endometriosis but none, at this time, can stand in place of laparoscopy.

REFERENCES

1. Houston, D.E., Noller, R.L., Melton, L.J. and Selwyn, B.J. (1987). Incidence of pelvic endometriosis in Rochester, Minnesota. *Am. J. Epidemiol.*, **125**, 959–69

2. Djursing, H., Petersen, K. and Weberg, E. (1981). Symptomatic postmenopausal endometriosis. *Acta. Obstet. Gynecol. Scand.*, **60**, 529

3. Wheeler, J.M. (1989). Epidemiology of endometriosis-associated infertility. *J. Reprod. Med.*, **34**, 41–6

4. Pauerstein, C.J. (1989). Clinical presentation and diagnosis. In Schenken, R.S. (ed). *Endometriosis. Contemporary Concepts in Clinical Management.* pp. 127–44. (Philadelphia: Lippincott).

5. Scott, R.B. and Te Linde, R.W. (1950). External endometriosis: the scourge of the private patient. *Ann. Surg.*, **131**, 706

6. Jenkins, S., Olive, D.L. and Haney, A.F.(1986). Endometriosis: pathogenic implications of the anatomic distribution. *Obstet. Gynecol.*, **67**, 335–8

7. O'Connor, D.T. (1987). *Endometriosis.* (Edinburgh: Churchill Livingstone)

8. Portuando, J.A., Herrciu, C., Echanogarrengni, A.D. and Reigo, A.G. (1982). Peritoneal flushing and biopsy in laparoscopically diagnosed endometriosis. *Fertil. Steril.*, **38**, 538

9. Vasquez, G., Cornillie, F. and Brosens, I. (1984). Peritoneal endometriosis: scanning electron microscopy and histology of minimal pelvic endometriotic lesions. *Fertil. Steril.*, **42**, 696–703

10. Murphy, A.A., Green, W.R., Bobbie, D., de la Cruz, Z.C. and Rock, J.A. (1986). Unsuspected endometriosis documented scanning electron microscopy in visually normal peritoneum. *Fertil. Steril.*, **46**, 522–4

11. Redwine, D.B. (1987). Age-related evolution in colour appearance of endometriosis. *Fertil. Steril.*, **48**, 1062–3

12. Jansen, R.P.S. and Russell, P. (1986). Nonpigmented endometriosis: clinical, laparoscopic, and pathological definition. *Am. J. Obstet. Gynecol.*, **155**, 1154–9

13. Brosens. I., Vasquez, G. and Gordts, S. (1984). Scanning electron microscopy study of the pelvic peritoneum in unexplained infertility and endometriosis. *Fertil. Steril.*, **42**, 218

14. Vernon, M.W., Beard, J.S., Graves, K. and Wilson, E.A. (1986). Classification of endometriotic implants by morphologic appearance and capacity to synthesize prostaglandin F. *Fertil. Steril.*, **46**, 801–6

15. Bast, R.C., Feeney, M., Lazarus, H., Nadler, L.M., Colvin, R.B. and Knapp, R.C. (1981). Reactivity of a monoclonal antibody with human ovarian carcinoma. *J. Clin. Invest.*, **68**, 1331

16. Barbieri, R.L. Niloff, J.M., Blast, R.C., Shaetzl, E., Kistner, R.W. and Knapp, R.C. (1986). Elevated serum concentrations of CA-125 in patients with advanced endometriosis. *Fertil. Steril.*, **45**, 630–4

17. Patton, P.E., Field, C.S. Harms, R.W. and Coulam, C.B. (1986). CA-125 levels in endometriosis. *Fertil. Steril.*, **45**, 770–2

18. Pittaway, D.E. and Douglas, J.W. (1989). Serum CA-125 in women with endometriosis and chronic pelvic pain. *Fertil. Steril.*, **51**, 68–70

19. Kennedy, S.H., Brodrib, J. and Barlow, D.H. (1988). Serum CA-125 changes after medical treatment for endometriosis. *Human Reproduction*, Suppl 1, **3**, 20

20. Williams, R.S., Venkateswara, C. and Yussman, M.A. (1988). Interference in the measurement of CA-125 in peritoneal fluid. *Fertil. Steril.*, **49**, 547–50

21. Fedele, L., Vercellini, P., Arcaini, L., da Dalt, M.G. and Candiani, G.B. (1988). CA-125 in serum, peritoneal fluid, active lesions, and endometrium of patients with endometriosis. *Am. J. Obstet. Gynecol.*, **158**, 166–70

22. Gleicher, N., El-Roeiy, A., Confino, E. and Friberg, J. (1987). Is endometriosis an autoimmune disease? *Obstet. Gynecol.*, **70**, 115–122

23. Badawy, S.Z.A., Cuenca, V., Stitzel, A., Jacobs, R.D.B., and Tomar, R.H. (1984). Autoimmune phenomena in infertile patients with endometriosis. *Obstet. Gynecol.*, **63**, 271

24. Mathur, S., Peress, M.R., Williamson, H.O., Youmans, C.D., Maney, S.A., Garvey, A.J., Rust, P.F. and Fudenberg, H.H. (1982). Autoimmunity to endometrium and ovary in endometriosis. *Clin. Exp. Immunol.*, **50**, 259.

25. Chihal, H.J., Mathur, S., Holtz, G.L. and Williamson, H.O. (1986). An antiendometrial antibody assay in the clinical diagnosis and management of endometriosis. *Fertil. Steril.*, **46**, 408–11

26. Kennedy, S.H., Sargent, P.M., Hicks, B.R. and Barlow, D.H. (1989). Immunohistochemical detection of anti-endometrial antibodies. (Abstract). *2nd International Symposium on Endometriosis*. p. 26 (Houston, Texas)

27. Moncayo, R. and Moncayo-Naveda, H. (1989). Human autoantibodies against endometrium in patients with endometriosis; development of an enzyme immunoassay. (abstract). *J. Reprod. Immunol.*, Suppl., p. 191

28. Starkey, P., Kennedy, S., Sargent, I., Hicks, B., and Barlow, D. (1989). An enzyme linked immunabsorbant assay for antiendometrial antibodies.

(abstract). *J. Reprod. Immunol.*, Suppl., 190

29. Friedman, H., Vogelsang, R.L., Mendelson, E.B., Neiman, H.L. and Cohen, M. (1985). Endometriosis detection by US with laparoscopic correlation. *Radiology*, **157**, 217–20

30. Kennedy, S.H., Brodribb, J., Godfrey, A.M. and Barlow, D.H. (1988). Pre-operative treatment of an abdominal wall endometrioma with nafarelin acetate. Case report. *Br. J. Obstet. Gynaecol.*, **95**, 521–3

31. Johnson, I.R., Symonds, E.M., Worthington, B.S., Kean, D.M., Johnson, J., Gyngell, M. and Hawkes, R.C. (1984). Imaging ovarian tumours by nuclear magnetic imaging. *Br. J. Obstet. Gynaecol.*, **91**, 260–4.

32. Dooms, G.C., Hricak, H. and Tscholakoff, D. (1986). Adnexal structures: MR imaging. *Radiology*, **158**, 639–46

33. Butler, H., Bryan, P.I., Lipuma, J.R., Cohen, A.M., El Yousef, S., Andriole, J.G. and Lieberman, J. (1984). Magnetic resonance imaging of the abnormal female pelvis. *Am. J. Radiol.*, **143**, 1259–66

34. Kennedy, S.H. Soper, N.D.W., Mojiminiyi, O.A., Shepstone, B.J. and Barlow, D.H. (1988). Immunoscintigraphy of ovarian endometriosis. A preliminary study. *Br. J. Obstet. Gynaecol.*, **95**, 693–7

DISCUSSION

Prof. Shaw

Many of our colleagues, and certainly our junior staff, are not aware of the subtle changes of endometriosis, so the disease is being underdiagnosed. Also there has been some evidence that if one looks at serum levels of CA-125 there is quite a good correlation with the degree of peritoneal adhesions. Is this perhaps reflecting itself with the immunoscintigraphy results in that adhesions are being identified and perhaps the marker is picking some other expression of peritoneal inflammation?

Mr Barlow

That is very reasonable. Gynaecological practice does vary throughout Europe. If we had a technique which would even allow us to say that this patient has some form of peritoneal disease process going on, this would be useful in itself and help identify who to investigate further.

2

Endometriosis: pathogenesis and pathophysiology

J. Donnez, M. Nisolle, F. Casanas-Roux and P. Grandjean

INTRODUCTION

The term endometriosis is defined pathologically by the presence of tissue outside the uterus that is histologically similar to endometrium. Endometrial tissue within the myometrium termed adenomyosis is a separate pathological entity with a different patient population, aetiology, and clinical course[1].

Endometriosis is very accurately diagnosed by visual inspection of the pelvis, and histological confirmation is not mandatory for clinical decision making. Pathologists have required the presence of glands, stroma, and evidence of menstrual cyclicity (tissue haemorrhage or haemosiderin-laden macrophages) to make the diagnosis categorically. But ectopically-implanted endometrium rarely has the identical microscopic appearance or architecture of normal endometrium *in situ*. The implants are composed of isolated scattered glandular and stromal components rather than exact copies of intrauterine endometrium, because menstrual shedding of endometrium occurs as isolated cells rather than intact fragments of endometrium[1].

For the purpose of this chapter, endometriosis will be defined by the presence of endometrial glands and stroma, with or without evidence of menstrual cyclicity (haemosiderin-laden macrophages), outside the uterus.

PATHOGENESIS

Van Rokitansky provided the first detailed description of endometriosis in 1860[2], and many theories of pathogenesis have been put forward since that time. Endometriosis is a unique disease process characterized by its invasive but non-neoplastic growth pattern, the presence of endometrium at ectopic sites, and evidence of hormonal responsiveness with menstrual cyclicity.

Transplantation

In the course of a series of publications, J.A. Sampson proposed a theory for the development of endometriosis[3-7]. He observed that "the menstrual effluent contained viable endometrial cells of both the stromal and glandular elements, which could be transplanted to ectopic sites by retrograde menstruation" i.e. through the Fallopian tubes. Several other routes of dissemination have been observed including lymphatic, vascular and iatrogenic dissemination. Retrograde menstruation through the Fallopian tubes probably represents the route of dissemination in the majority of patients whose disease is confined to the peritoneal surface of the pelvic peritoneum.

Retrograde Menstruation
After observing the pattern of endometriosis for many years, Sampson concluded that endometrial cells regurgitated through the Fallopian tubes at the time of menstruation explained the vast majority of endometriosis he observed.

To understand the retrograde menstrual process, the physiology of the normal menstrual cycle must be well understood. In virtually all mammalian species, cyclical ovarian changes culminating in ovulation occur. In most animals, coitus or the presence of a conceptus is required to develop a luteal phase. In human and sub-human primates, spontaneous luteal phases occur in the absence of coitus or a conceptus. Functional changes in the endometrium, i.e. secretory endometrium with decidualisation and biochemical events necessary to prepare the genital tract for early embryo growth, occur in response to progesterone secreted by the corpus luteum.

In the case of pregnancy, human chorionic gonadotrophin (hCG), provides trophic support to the corpus luteum. In the absence of a conceptus, the corpus luteum undergoes a regression, which provokes a reduction in progesterone production and menses which involves a shedding of endometrial cells with tissue fluid and blood[1,8].

Uterine prostaglandin production is intimately involved with menstruation[9]. Endometrial tissue gains the ability to synthesize prostaglandins late in the luteal phase. Vasoconstricting prostaglandins cause a spasm of the spiral arterioles supplying the superficial layers of endometrium; tissue hypoxia and ischaemia are the consequence. Blood, extra-cellular fluid and cells are shed and comprise the menstrual effluent[1,8]. Examinations of the cellular content demonstrate that the cell loss is predominantly of individual cells rather than intact fragments of endometrium.

Prostaglandins provoke myometrial contractions and a high intrauterine pressure[1,9]. There are three possible routes of egress for the menstrual effluent: the cervix and each of the Fallopian tubes. The greatest volume of menstrual flow goes through the cervical canal which has a larger diameter than the oviducts. The utero-tubal junction probably prevents regurgitation of menstrual debris, under the influence of prostaglandins.

Three criteria must be met to allow consideration of retrograde menstruation as the explanation for pathogenesis of pelvic endometriosis. First, endometrial cells must enter the peritoneal cavity through the Fallopian tubes. Secondly, cells within the menstrual debris must be viable, and able to be transplanted on pelvic structures. Thirdly, the anatomical distribution of endometriosis in the pelvic cavity must be correlated with the principles of transplantation for exfoliated cells[10].

The entry of viable endometrial cells through the Fallopian tubes was proved as follows:

(1)   The presence of endometrial cells has been demonstrated in the Fallopian tube[11] and in the peritoneal cavity by cytological evaluation of peritoneal fluid[12,13].

(2)   Retrograde menstruation has been demonstrated to occur universally. Some menstrual regurgitation must occur almost universally, as evidenced by bloody peritoneal dialysates at the time

of menses[14] and haemorrhagic peritoneal fluid retrieved at laparoscopy during menses[15–17].

The viability of endometrial cells and the ability of them to be transplanted was proved by:

(1) Presence of viable endometrial cells in the menses has been demonstrated by culturing the menstrual effluent and obtaining tissue cultures of endometrial cells.

(2) Endometrial cells obtained from the menstrual effluent have been demonstrated to be transplantable to abdominal wall fascia[18].

(3) Endometriosis can be induced by implantation of endometrial tissue[19,20].

(4) Oestrogen and progesterone are not required for implantation of endometrial cells, but do maintain viable endometrial implants[21].

The principles of transplantation for exfoliated cells are as outlined:

(1) The tubal ostia are located near the uterosacral ligament in Douglas' pouch which is one of the most common sites of endometrial cell implantation[22].

(2) Transplantation of free-floating endometrial cells in the peritoneal cavity appears to be influenced by the effects of gravity. Indeed endometriosis is rarely observed in the upper abdominal peritoneal cavity[22].

(3) Endometrial implantation occurs less often in mobile pelvic structures such as the Fallopian tubes and the small bowel than in fixed structures such as the ovaries, the pelvic peritoneum and the fixed portion of the sigmoid colon[22].

(4) The type of surface epithelium, vascularity, and hormone production could influence transplantation production. The epithelium lining the lower genital tract is poorly vascularised whereas the peritoneum overlying the pelvic viscera has good vascularisation. Ovarian hormone production is necessary for growth, and high concentration of ovarian steroids has been

observed in the peritoneal fluid of women with ovulatory cycles[23,24]. The ovary is an optimal site for implantation because of the proximity to the tubal ostia, the poor vascularisation for the ovarian capsule and high intraovarian steroid concentrations[10,22,25,26].

To explain why endometriosis occurs in just 1–2% of women, whereas regurgitation occurs probably in all women during their reproductive years, other factors must be considered. The first could be the volume of regurgitated debris. When no significant pathology exists, the pressure relationships between the cervix and Fallopian tubes is likely to determine the proportion of menses that is regurgitated, but little is known of the determinants of directional flow of menstrual effluent. Interestingly, women with short cycle lengths and menses for a week or longer have been reported to have greater than twice the risk of developing endometriosis. Aetiological factors such as heredity contribution and immunological deficiency are probably the explanation for implantation.

Lymphatic and haematogenous dissemination
To explain the presence of endometriosis outside the peritoneal cavity, other ways of dissemination have been suggested. Lymphatic drainage of endometrial cells was first suggested by Halbin[27], and Sampson[5] suggested vascular transport as a route of dissemination of endometrium to distant sites. The presence of endometrial tissue within lymphatic channels, lymph nodes[28–30] and pelvic veins[31] has now been established.

Iatrogenic dissemination
Implantation of endometrial cells at the time of surgery has been considered in publications by numerous gynaecologists, from laparotomy to episiotomy as the explanations of endometrial deposits within surgical scars[18].

Coelomic metaplasia

Another theory regarding the development of the disease is the theory of coelomic metaplasia, as described by Meyer[32]. This theory explains the development of endometriosis by differentiation (by metaplasia) of the original coelomic membrane into the endometrial glands and stroma.

Many reports support this theory:

(1) Endometriosis has been reported in the prostatic utricle of men with prostatic carcinoma undergoing high-dose oestrogen therapy[33,34].

(2) Cases of "Müllerian agenesis" have been associated with endometriosis. Typically, the Fallopian tubes are present, as well as a small blind uterine horn at the medial portion of the tube providing the source of endometrial cells[35].

(3) In some cases of Rokintanski–Kuster–Hauser syndrome, endometriosis has also been described. In this syndrome, there is no endometrium capable of being a source of endometriotic cells, which must have developed *de novo*.

There are also data which do not support this theory. If metaplasia represents the pathophysiological process, the distribution on the peritoneal surface would be uniform and increase with age. However:

(a) endometriotic implants are not uniformly distributed within the peritoneum;

(b) the coelomic membrane contributes both to the peritoneal cavity and the lining of the thoracic cavity[36,37], but endometriosis has rarely been reported in the chest;

(c) endometriosis is confined to women in the reproductive years and is abruptly halted by the decrease in gonadal hormones at the climacteric. There is no proof that the metaplasia is an oestrogen-induced process.

Considering the above arguments, it might be considered that the coelomic metaplasia theory for development of endometriosis has virtually no supporting scientific evidence and appears to be of historical interest only. Recently, however, some data lead to demonstration that the coelomic membrane can undergo metaplasia in the adult. Indeed, during the last decade, a few authors[38–42] have hinted at the subtle variety of appearance of peritoneal endometriosis. Some of these data suggested the possibility of a biological continuum between non-pigmented and pigmented endometriotic lesions[38]. In some cases, they proved their hypothesis by a second-look laparoscopy: the non-pigmented lesions left untreated during the first laparoscopy progressed to typical pigmented lesions – this is an argument in favour of the coelomic metaplasia theory.

Embryonic rests of Müllerian origin

Another possible aetiology is the stimulation of embryonic rests of Müllerian origin. The anatomical distribution of endometriosis, however, does not follow the path of the Müllerian (paramesonephric) duct system and consequently there is virtually nothing to support that concept.

Conclusion

Endometriosis is probably a consequence of transplantation of viable endometrial cells regurgitated through the Fallopian tubes at the time of menses. However, the dissemination of viable endometrial cells can occur by other routes and some cases can only be explained by the metaplasia theory.

PATHOLOGY: PERITONEAL ENDOMETRIOSIS SUBTLE APPEARANCES

Endometriosis most commonly affects the pelvic peritoneum close to the ovaries, including the uterosacral ligaments, the ovarian fossa peritoneum, and the peritoneum of the cul-de-sac.

The increased diagnosis of endometriosis at laparoscopy can be explained by the increased ability to detect such subtle lesions through the surgeon's experience (in our own hospital the diagnosis of endometriosis at laparoscopy increased from 42% in 1982 to 72% in 1988). The greatest change was in the case of "subtle" lesions, which increased from 15% in 1986 to 65% in 1988. The diagnosis of peritoneal endometriosis at the time of laparoscopy is often made by observation of typically puckered black or bluish lesions. There are in addition the numerous subtle appearances of peritoneal endometriosis. These lesions, frequently non-pigmented, were diagnosed as endometriosis following biopsy confirmation by Jansen and Russell in 1986[38,40,43].

Table 1   Different appearances of peritoneal endometriosis

Typical aspect
  Puckered black lesion

Subtle lesions
  White opacification (Jansen and Russell[38], 1986)
  Red flamelike lesion (Jansen[38], 1986)
  Glandular excrescences (Jansen[38], 1986)
  Subovarian adhesions (Jansen[38], 1986)
  Yellow–brown peritoneal patches (Jansen[38], 1986)
  Circular peritoneal defect (Chatman[44], 1981)
  Petechial peritoneum (Donnez and Nisolle[42], 1988)
  Hypervascularization areas (Donnez and Nisolle[42], 1988)

Typical lesion

The typical peritoneal endometriotic lesion results from tissue bleeding and retention of blood pigment producing brown discolouration of tissue. Puckered black lesions are a combination of glands, stroma, scar and intraluminal debris. The macroscopic appearance of ectopic endometrium is probably dependent upon the longevity of the process. Viable cells may implant and the initial appearance may be an irregularity or discolouration of the peritoneal surface – the earliest sign being haemosiderin staining of the peritoneal surfaces. Initially, these lesions may appear haemorrhagic, but menstrual shedding from a viable endometrial implant initiates an inflammatory reaction which provokes a scarification process which in turn encloses the implants. The presence of entrapped 'menstrual debris is responsible for the typical black or bluish appearance. If the inflammatory process obliterates or devascularises the endometrial cells, eventually this discolouration disappears. A white plaque of old collagen is all that remains of the ectopic implant.

Scarring of the peritoneum around endometrial implants is a typical finding. In addition to encapsulating an isolated implant, the scar may deform the surrounding peritoneum or result in the development of adhesions between adjacent pelvic viscera. Pelvic adhesions due to endometriosis are most common between the immobile pelvic structures which are in natural apposition within the pelvic cavity. Adhesions caused by endometriosis are commonly found between the posterior leaf of the broad ligament and the ovary and between the dependent sigmoid colon and the posterior aspect of the vagina and the cervix.

Subtle appearance
Sometimes the subtle endometriotic lesions can be the only lesions seen at laparoscopy[40,41,43]. These subtle forms are more common and may be more active and more important than the puckered black lesions. The non-pigmented endometriotic peritoneal lesions include the following.

(1)   White opacification of the peritoneum which appears as peritoneal scarring or as circumscribed patches, often thickened and sometimes raised. Histologically, white opacified peritoneum is due to the presence of an occasional retroperitoneal glandular structure and scanty stroma surrounded by fibrotic tissue or connective tissue.

(2)   Red flame-like lesions of the peritoneum or red vesicular excrescences affect more commonly the broad ligament and the uterosacral ligaments. Histologically, red flame-like lesions and vesicular excrescences are due to the presence of active endometriosis surrounded by stroma.

(3)   Glandular excrescences on the peritoneal surface which in colour, translucency and consistency closely resemble the mucosal surface of the endometrium seen at hysteroscopy. Biopsy reveals the presence of numerous endometrial glands.

(4)   Subovarian adhesions or adherence between ovary and peritoneum of the ovarian fossa which are distinctive from adhesions characteristic of previous salpingitis or peritonitis. Histologically, connective tissue with sparse endometrial glands were found.

(5)   Yellow-brown peritoneal patches resembling *café au lait* patches. These often affect the cul de sac, the broad ligament or the bladder. The histological characteristics are similar to those observed in white opacification, but in the yellow-brown patches the presence of the blood pigment – haemosiderin – amongst the stroma cells produces the *café au lait* colour.

(6)　Circular peritoneal defects as described by Chatman[44]. These are defects in the pelvic peritoneum on the uterosacral ligament or the broad ligament. Serial section will demonstrate the presence of endometrial glands in more than 50% of cases.

(7)　Areas of petechial peritoneum or areas with hypervascularisation were diagnosed as endometriosis in our recent study[45]. Moreover, Goldstein and colleagues[46] documented petechial and blood-like endometriosis as the only finding in 20% of their adolescent patients. These lesions resemble the petechial lesion due to manipulation of peritoneum or to hypervascularisation of peritoneum. They most generally affect the bladder and the broad ligament, and histologically, red blood cells are numerous and endometrial glands are very rare.

Histological study of peritoneal endometriosis

The morphological characteristics of peritoneal endometriosis were studied in 109 biopsies with histologically proved endometriosis (Table 2). An endometriotic lesion was considered "active" when typical glandular epithelium appeared as either proliferative or completely unresponsive to hormones, with typical stroma. Such a lesion was found in 76% of cases. Areas of oviduct-like epithelium with ciliated cells were demonstrated in 55% of peritoneal endometriotic foci. The epithelial height and the mitotic index were calculated in typical glandular epithelium. Epithelial height was measured with a micrometer and the mitotic index was calculated by counting mitotic figures per 2000 epithelial cells, as previously described[16,47]. Their value was respectively $14.8 \pm 3.2 \, \mu m$ and 0.6‰.

Brown and black colouration appears to be a function of the amount of intraluminal haemosiderin and debris. The dark, pigmented stigmas that compose the usual visual criteria for diagnosis of endometriosis are the late consequence of this cyclic growth and regression of the lesions, to the point where tissue bleeding and discolouration by blood pigment have taken place. In the absence of conspicuous occurence of blood pigment, diagnosis of endometriosis is likely to be missed. Confirmation of endometriosis in subtle lesions was performed by Jansen and Russell[38].

Table 2 Morphological characteristics in peritoneal endometriosis

Biopsies	n = *109*
Typical glandular epithelium and stroma	109 (100%)
Active endometriosis	83 (76%)
Oviduct-like epithelium	46 (55%)
Epithelial height (μm)	14.8 ± 3.2
Mitotic index (‰)	0.6

Endometriosis was confirmed in 81% of white opacified lesions, 81% of red flame-like lesions, 67% of glandular lesions, 50% of subovarian adhesions, 47% of yellow-brown patches and 45% of circular peritoneal defects. Later, Stripling and colleagues[40] confirmed endometriosis in 91% of white lesions, 75% of red lesions, 33% of haemosiderin lesions, and 85% of other lesions. In our study[45], we confirmed the presence of endometriotic lesions in non-pigmented lesions of peritoneum in more than 50% of cases. The ability to detect subtle endometriotic lesions must be an advantage all gynaecologists possess. Indeed, such lesions must be detected, because they are probably the first stage of peritoneal endometriosis and afford explanation of further development of the disease.

Endometriosis in macroscopically normal peritoneum

Unsuspected peritoneal endometriosis
This can be found in the visually normal peritoneum of infertile women with associated endometriosis or it can be missed. Identification of endometriosis in biopsy specimens from areas of normal peritoneum in patients with known endometriosis was reported by Murphy and colleagues[48].

By scanning electron microscopy, 25% of their specimens that appeared normal by gross inspection were found to contain evidence of endometriosis. By light microscopy, an incidence of 13% was reported in our study[45], biopsies being taken from a visually normal peritoneum, contiguous with a pigmented lesion or with areas of subtle appearances of peritoneal endometriosis. When taking biopsies from visually normal peritoneum in infertile women without any typical or subtle endometriotic lesions, our histological study revealed the presence of endometriosis in 6% of cases. This suggests that the absence of endometriosis in infertile women must be confirmed by biopsy from uterosacral ligament peritoneum.

PATHOLOGY: OVARIAN ENDOMETRIOSIS

The ovary represents a relatively unique site of implantation, as the levels of gonadal steroids surpass those in the circulation, and hence this affords an ideal environment for implantation and endometrial growth. Superficial implants of endometriosis on the ovary resemble implants at other peritoneal sites. In contrast, when endometrial cells enter the ovarian stroma, large endometrial cysts may form that are filled with a viscous chocolate-coloured liquid, i.e. "chocolate cysts" or endometrioma, which represent debris from cyclic menstruation[3]. There is usually a well demarcated separation between the endometrial cyst wall and the normal adjacent ovarian stroma. The epithelial lining of the endometrioma may initially have resembled the endometrium, but with continued menstrual cyclicity without drainage of the menstrual material, pressure atrophy compresses the epithelium into a flat cuboidal pattern without specific distinguishing characteristics.

The entry of endometrial cells into the ovarian stroma has long been a source of controversy. It has been suggested that the ovulatory stigma represents an optimal site for implantation, because it marks a break in the ovarian capsule. This hypothesis is wholly in opposition to that of Koninckx and colleagues[12] who suggested that the absence of stigma (LUF syndrome) is responsible for implantation of endometrial cells in the peritoneal cavity.

Secretory function of endometrial implants and hormonal responsiveness to hormonal therapy

Using qualitative histochemistry, the microscopic changes present in endometrium have been observed in ectopic implants[49], but endometrial implants do not demonstrate the characteristic ultrastructural changes of normal endometrium[50]. Prostanoid concentrations in the peritoneal fluid of women with endometriosis have been found to be elevated[51,52], but other studies have not confirmed these observations[53,54]. Prostaglandins are also synthesized by peritoneal macrophages.

The fact that endometrial implants can undergo cyclical histological changes similar to those found with normal endometrium demonstrates that ectopic endometrium responds to gonadal hormones. But the majority of implants do not demonstrate synchronous histological changes with the comparable uterine endometrium[55]. Among the reasons are probably:

(1) deficiency in steroid receptors,

(2) the influence of the surrounding scarification process,

(3) pressure atrophy,

(4) the hormonal independence of ectopic endometrial glands.

The evaluation of steroid receptors in ectopic endometrial implants could be difficult because of the small number of glandular and stromal cells within the implant, and the heterogeneity of the tissue. While most implants can be demonstrated to possess progesterone receptors, only 30% have oestrogen receptors[56]. On the ovary, implants have far fewer oestrogen and progesterone receptors than does normal epithelium[57,58]. Castration, menopause, pregnancy or therapeutic suppression of gonadal function can dramatically alter the pattern of disease. We have recently shown (Nisolle and colleagues) that hormonal treatment is unable to eradicate endometriosis[47]. Since both in peritoneal endometriosis and in ovarian endometriosis, microscopic examination of specimens (taken after 6 months of therapy) revealed a high incidence of active endometriosis without signs of degeneration[47]. Mitotic activity was found, and this suggested the presence of hormonal independent glands in endometriotic foci.

In ongoing work we have evaluated the DNA content in the nucleus of glandular cells from peritoneal and ovarian endometriosis in women without hormonal therapy or after hormonal therapy. The DNA content was similar in all groups, suggesting the nuclear activity and the RNA synthesis were not modified although a suppressive therapy was being administered.

Conclusion

There is a substantial variability in the histological appearance of ectopic endometrium.

The exact reason why a number of implants or cells do not respond to hormonal therapy is not known, but at least three hypotheses have been proposed.

(1) Endometriotic cells may have their own genetic programming, while endocrine influence appears to be only secondary and dependent on the degree of differentiation of the individual cell.

(2) The low number of endometriotic steroid receptors and their differing regulatory mechanisms in ectopic and eutopic endometrium may result in deficient endocrine dependency.

(3) The scarification process surrounding the implants may modify the vascularisation.

REFERENCES

1. Flowers, C.E. Jr. and Wilborn, W.H. (1978). New observations in the physiology of menstruation. *Obstet.Gynecol.*, **51**, 16–24
2. Ridley, J.H. (1968). The histogenesis of endometriosis: a review of facts and fancies. *Obstet. Gynecol. Survey*, **23**, 1–25
3. Sampson, J.A. (1921). Perforating hemorrhagic (chocolate) cysts of the ovary. *Arch.Surgery*, **3**, 245–323
4. Sampson, J.A. (1924). Benign and malignant endometrial implants in the peritoneal cavity and their relation to certain ovarian tumors. *Surg. Gynecol. Obstet.*, **38**, 287
5. Sampson, J.A. (1925). Heterotopic or misplaced endometrial tissue. *Am. J. Obstet. Gynecol.*, **10**, 649–64
6. Sampson, J.A. (1927). Peritoneal endometriosis due to dissemination of endometrial tissue into the peritoneal cavity. *Am. J. Obstet. Gynecol.*, **14**, 422–69
7. Sampson, J.A. (1945). Pathogenesis of postsalpingectomy endometriosis in laparotomy scars. *Am. J. Obstet. Gynecol.*, **59**, 596–620
8. Markee, J.E. (1948). Morphological basis for menstrual bleeding. *Bull. NY Acad. Med.*, **24**, 253–68
9. Vijayakumar, R. and Walters, W.A.W. (1981). Myometrial prostaglandins

during the human menstrual cycle. *Am. J. Obstet. Gynecol.*, **141**, 313

10. Holmes, W.R. (1980). Endometriosis: associations with menorrhagia, infertility and oral contraceptives. *Int. J. Gynecol. Obstet.*, **17**, 573

11. Geist, S.H. (1979). The viability of fragments of menstrual endometrium. *Am. J. Obstet. Gynecol.*, **25**, 751

12. Manning, J.O. and Shaver, E.F. Jr. (1959). The demonstration of endometrial cells by Papanicolaou and supravital techniques obtained by culdocentesis. *Bull. Tulane Univ. Med. Fac.*, **18**, 193

13. Koninckx, P.R., Ide, P., Vandenbroucke, W. and Brosens, I.A. (1980). New aspects of the pathophysiology of endometriosis and associated infertility. *J. Reprod. Med.*, **24**, 257–60

14. Blumenkrantz, M.J., Gallagher, N., Bashore, R.A. *et al.* (1981). Retrograde menstruation in women undergoing chronic peritoneal dialysis. *Obstet. Gynecol.*, **57**, 667–70

15. Halme, J., Hammond, M.G., Hulka, J.F. *et al.* (1984). Retrograde menstruation in healthy women and in patients with endometriosis. *Obstet. Gynecol.*, **64**, 151–54

16. Liu, D.T.Y. and Hitchcock, A. (1986). Endometriosis: its association with retrograde menstruation, dysmenorrhea and tubal pathology. *Br. J. Obstet. Gynecol.*, **93**, 859–62

17. Donnez, J., Langerock, S. and Thomas, K. (1981). Environment hormonal intra-abdominal de l'utérus chez la femme. In Colloque de la Société Nationale pour l'étude de la stérilité et de la fécondité. Utérus et fécondité. 1981, p.83. (Paris: Masson)

18. Ridley, J.H. and Edwards, I.K. (1958). Experimental endometriosis in the human. *Am. J. Obstet. Gynecol.*, **76**, 783–90

19. Allen, E., Peterson, L.F. and Campbell, Z.B. (1954). Clinical and experimental endometriosis. *Am. J. Obstet. Gynecol.*, **68**, 356–75

20. Schencken, R.Q., Asch, R.H., Williams, R.F. and Hodgen, G.D. (1984). Etiology of infertility in monkeys with endometriosis: luteinized unruptured follicles, luteal phase defects, pelvic adhesions, and spontaneous abortions. *Fertil. Steril.*, **41**, 122–30

21. Dizeraga, G.S., Barber, D.L. and Hodgen, G.D. (1980). Endometriosis: role of ovarian steroids in initiation, maintenance and suppression. *Fertil. Steril.*, **33**, 649–60

22. Jenkins, S., Olive, D.L. and Haney, A.F. (1986). Endometriosis: pathogenetic implications of the anatomic distribution. *Obstet. Gynecol.*, **67**, 335–8

23. Koninckx, P.R., De Moor, P. and Brosens, I.A. (1980). Diagnosis of the luteinized unruptured follicle syndrome by steroid hormone assay on peritoneal fluid. *Br. J. Obstet. Gynaecol.*, **87**, 929–34

24. Donnez, J., Langerock, S. and Thomas, K. (1983). Peritoneal fluid volume, 17 beta-estradiol and progresterone concentrations in women with endometriosis and/or luteinized unruptured follicle syndrome. *Gynecol. Obstet. Invest.*, **16**, 210–20

25. Scott, R.B. and Te Linde, R.W. (1950). External endometriosis: scourge of the private patient. *Ann. Surg.*, **131**, 697–720

26. Haney, A.F., Handwerger, S. and Weiberg, J.B. (1984). Peritoneal fluid prolactin in infertile women with endometriosis: lack of evidence of secretory activity by endometric implants. *Fertil. Steril.*, **42**, 935–8

27. Halbin, J. (1925). Hysoticteroadenosis metastatica, Die lymphogere genese der sog, Adenofibromatis heterotopica. *Arch. Gynack.*, **124**, 457

28. Javert, C.T. (1949). Pathogenesis of endometriosis based on endometrial homeoplasia direct extension, exfoliation and implantation, lymphomatic and hematogeneous metastasis. *Cancer*, **2**, 399–410

29. Koss, I.G. (1963). Miniature adenocanthoma arising in an adenometriotic cyst in an obturator lymph node. *Cancer*, **16**, 1369–72

30. Scott, R.B., Novak, R.J. and Tindale, R.M. (1958). Umbilical endometriosis and Cullen's sign: study of lymphatic transport from pelvis to umbilicus in monkeys. *Obset. Gynecol.*, **11**, 556–63

31. Javert, C.T. (1952). The spread of benign and malignant endometrium in the lymphatic system with a note of coexisting vascular involvement. *Am. J. Obstet. Gynecol.*, **64**, 780–806

32. Meyer, R. (1919). Uber den Staude der Frage der Adenomyosites Adenomyoma in Allgemeinen und Adenomyonetitis Sarcomastosa. *Zent. Fur. Gynack.*, **36**, 745–59

33. Melicow, M.M. and Pachter, M.R. (1967). Endometrial carcinoma of the prostatic utricle (uterus masculinus). *Cancer*, **20**, 1715–22

34. Schrodt, G.R. Alcorn, M.D. and Ibanez, J. (1980). Endometriosis of the male urinary system: a case report. *J. Urol.*, **124**, 722–23

35. Rosenfeld, D.L. and Lecher, B.D. (1981). Endometriosis in a patient with Rokitansky–Kuster–Hauser syndrome. *Am. J. Obstet. Gynecol.*, **139**, 105

36. Maximow, A. (1927). Uber der Mesthel (Deckzellen der serosen Haute) und die Zellen der sero sen Exsudate. Utersuchungen an entzundetem Gewebe und and Gewebskulturen. *Arch. Exp. Zellforch.*, **4**, 1

37. Filatow, D. (1933). Uber die Bildung des Anfangsstaddiums bie der Extremitatenentwicklung. *Roux Arch fur Entwicklungsmechnd, Organe*, **127**, 776

38. Jansen, R.P.S. and Russell, P. (1986). Nonpigmented endometriosis: clinical laparoscopic and pathologic definition. *Am. J. Obstet. Gynecol.*, **155**, 1154–9

39. Redwine, D.B. (1987). The distribution of endometriosis in the pelvis by

age groups and fertility. *Fertil. Steril.*, **47**, 173–5

40. Stripling, M.C., Martin, D.C., Chatman, D.L. Vander Zwaag, R. and Poston, W.M. (1988). Subtle appearance of pelvic endometriosis. *Fertil. Steril.*, **49**, 427–31

41. Martin, D.C., Hubert, G.D., Vander Zwaag, R. and El-Zeky, F. (1989). Laparoscopic appearances of peritoneal endometriosis. *Fertil. Steril.*, **51**, 63–7

42. Donnez, J. and Nisolle, M. (1988). Appearance of peritoneal endometriosis. In *IIIrd Laser Surgery Symposium*. (Brussels)

43. Redwine, D.B. (1987). Age-related evolution in colour appearance of endometriosis. *Fertil. Steril.*, **47**, 1062–3

44. Chatman, D.L. (1981). Pelvic peritoneal defects and endometriosis; Allenmasters syndrome revisited. *Fertil. Steril.*, **36**, 751

45. Nisolle-Pochet, M., Paindaveine, B., Bourdon, A., Berlière, M., Casañas-Roux, F. and Donnez, J. (1989). Peritoneal endometriosis typical aspect and subtle appearance. *Fertil. Steril.* (In press)

46. Goldstein, D.P., de Cholnoky., Emans, S.J. and Leventhal, J.M. (1980). Laparoscopy in the diagnosis and management of pelvic pain in adolescents. *J. Reprod. Med.*, **24**, 251–6

47. Nisolle-Pochet, M., Casañas-Roux, F. and Donnez, J. (1988). Histologic study of ovarian endometriosis after hormonal therapy. *Fertil. Steril.*, **49**, 423–26

48. Murphy, A.A., Green, W.R., Bobbie, D., de la Cruz, Z.C. and Rock, J.A. (1986). Unsuspected endometriosis documented by scanning electron microscopy in visually normal peritoneum. *Fertil. Steril.*, **46**, 522–4

49. Brosens, I., Vasquez, G. and Gordts, S. (1984). Scanning electron microscopic study of the pelvic peritoneum in unexplained infertility and endometriosis. *Fertil. Steril.*, **41**, 215

50. Lox, C.D., Word, L., Heine, M.W. *et al.* (1984). Ultrastructural evaluation of endometriosis. *Fertil. Steril.*, **41**, 755

51. Meldrum, D., Shamonki, I. and Clark, K. (1977). Prostaglandin content of ascitic fluid in endometriosis: a preliminary report. Presented at the *25th Annual Meeting of the Pacific Coast Fertility Society*, Palm Springs, California.

52. Deleon, F.D., Vijayakumar, R., Brown, M., Rao, C.H.V., Yussman, M.A. and Schultz, G. (1986). Peritoneal fluid volume, estrogen, progesterone, prostaglandin, and epidermal growth factor concentrations in patients with and without endometriosis. *Obstet. Gynecol.*, **68**, 189–94

53. Rock, J.A., Dubin, N.H. and Ghodgaonkar, R.B. (1982). Cul-de-sac fluid in women with endometriosis: fluid volume and prostanoid concentration during the proliferative phase of the cycle-days 8 to 12. *Fertil. Steril.*, **37**, 747–50

54. Chacho, K.J., Chacho, S., Audresen, P.J. and Scommegma, A. (1986). Peritoneal fluid in patients with and without endometriosis: prostanoids and macrophages and their effect on the spermatozoa penetration assay. *Am. J. Obstet. Gynecol.*, **154**, 1290–9

55. Roddick, J.W., Conkey, G. and Jacobs, E.J. (1960). The hormonal response of endometriotic implants and its relationship to symptomatology. *Am. J. Obstet. Gynecol.*, **79**, 1173–7

56. Janne, O., Kauppila, A., Kokko, E. *et al.* (1981). Estrogen and progestin receptors in endometriosis lesions: comparison with endometrial tissue. *Am. J. Obstet. Gynecol.*, **141**, 562–6

57. Bergqvist, A., Rannevik, G., and Thorell, J. (1981). Estrogen and progesterone cytosol receptor concentration in endometriotic tissue and intrauterine endometrium. *Acta Obstet. Gynecol. Scand.*, **101** Suppl., 53–8

58. Tamaya, T., Motoyaha, T., Ohono, Y. *et al.* (1979). Steroid receptor levels and histology of endometriosis and adenomyosis. *Fertil. Steril.*, **31**, 396–400

DISCUSSION

Dr F. Cornillie
Using this new technique you need to analyze simultaneously the DNA of the implants and the endometrium to see whether the cells that survive having been implanted at ectopic sites are really doing something different from the ectopic cells. Is such work planned?

Prof. Donnez
These were preliminary results. We are now doing an evaluation of the DNA content in the endometrium and the endometrium implants of the same patient.

Prof. Shaw
The patients in whom there was a 10% incidence of endometriotic deposits from visually normal peritoneum, were these symptomatic patients presenting with pelvic pain, or were these just patients at random say having sterilization without symptoms?

Prof. Donnez
Only the group of patients with infertility. We have done a similar study in a group of women with pelvic pain in whom we found > 25%

endometrial glands and stroma.

Prof. Seppala

In view of the recent paper by David Liu from Nottingham who performed his laparoscopies and biopsies at the onset of menstruation and who claimed to find endometriosis in 100% of women, asymptomatic women, would Professor Donnez and his colleagues see differences if they were to time their laparoscopies or biopsies at different phases of the cycle?

Prof. Donnez

I cannot give an answer. In my department I perform all laparoscopies for infertility immediately post ovulation. I know that there are many reports describing the presence of endometrial cells in the peritoneal fluid taken from patients during menstruation, and diagnosis would then probably be difficult.

3

Deeply infiltrating pelvic endometriosis: a new entity

P.R. Koninckx and F.J. Cornillie

INTRODUCTION

Since its first description by Sampson[1], endometriosis has remained an enigmatic disease. Indeed, the aetiology, the natural history of the disease and the mechanisms of the associated infertility and/or pain are still not understood. Many hypotheses have been put forward, including retrograde menstruation[2], the luteinized unruptured follicle (LUF) syndrome[3], the immunological response[4] and the role of macrophages in peritoneal fluid[5], as well as metaplasia[6] and its induction[7]. Each hypothesis can explain some aspects; none, however, is able to explain all aspects of endometriosis, neither the exact mechanism(s) of the associated pain and/or infertility, nor the varieties of laparoscopic appearance.

Endometriosis has been known for a long time to occur as ovarian cysts (endometriomas) and sclerosing gunshot lesions in the pelvis. During the last few years, minimal endometriosis has been described as small vesicles and polypoid superficial lesions. Morphologically, these lesions generally were found to be active[8–10]. Since they occur more frequently in younger women[11], it was suggested that they are initial stages of endometriosis.

Deep, infiltrating endometriosis has been known clinically ever since hysterectomies were performed for pelvic pain and dyspareunia in women with nodular endometriosis in the rectovaginal septum, with or without bowel involvement. Only recently, by the introduction of the

CO_2 laser excisional techniques[12], a relatively high incidence of deep disease was also recognized in younger women[13].

As a consequence, a prospective study was set up to investigate systematically the depth of infiltration of endometriosis and its morphology.

MATERIALS AND METHODS

Patients

All women undergoing laparoscopy ($n = 243$) for infertility ($n = 147$), pelvic pain ($n = 78$) or both ($n = 18$), in the division of reproductive medicine between July, 1988 and August, 1989 were included in this study. The localization, the appearance, the width and the depth of infiltration were recorded for each endometriotic lesion. Some (superficial) lesions were vaporized, most were excised with the CO_2 laser (15 watt superpulse, 1060 Sharplan). The depth of infiltration was measured with a graded probe. These data were used to calculate the total area (cm^2) of pelvic endometriosis, and the total volume (cm^3) of endometriosis and the volume at different depths of infiltration. The ratio of the volume of endometriosis up to a certain depth of infiltration to the total volume was used to estimate the shape of the endometriotic lesion, i.e. a flat and superficial (ratio $\rightarrow 1$) versus a cylindrical and deep lesion (ratio $\rightarrow 0$). Endometriosis was scored according to the revised American Fertility Society (rAFS) classification system. Endometrial biopsies were taken with a Novak curette.

Assays

A blood sample was drawn before starting the laparoscopy, and peritoneal fluid was taken at the beginning of laparoscopy; both were then assayed for CA-125 (Centocor-kit). For the peritoneal fluid the assay had to be modified as follows: after sufficient serial dilutions in male serum, all peritoneal fluid samples became parallel with the standard curve (without hook effect), indicating that they could be assayed accurately.

MORPHOLOGY

Methods and criteria used have been described in detail elsewere[14]. Briefly, small lesions were fixed in 1.25% glutaraldehyde, embedded in Epon, processed for semithin (1 μm) sectioning and stained with toluidin blue. Larger lesions were fixed in buffered formalin, embedded in paraffin, and the 5 μm sections were stained with haematoxylin and eosin.

In those blocks cut perpendicularly to the peritoneal surface, the depth of infiltration was measured morphologically confirming the estimated depth during surgery ($r = 0.84$, $n = 15$). All specimens were studied by one of the authors (FC). Endometriosis was diagnosed only when endometrial glands and stroma were found, and biopsies were classified as active only when proliferation and/or secretion were seen.

Data analysis

Data were collected into DBASE III-plus database and processed with SAS using the paired and unpaired Student's *t*-test, the χ-square, Spearman correlation and anova.

RESULTS

Incidence and severity of endometriosis

Endometriosis was found in 71% of women presenting with infertility, in 83% of women with pelvic pain and in 78% of women with both complaints. According to the rAFS classification 34, 27, 28 and 10% of women with infertility, 41, 40, 14, and 5% of women with pelvic pain and 36, 29, 15 and 21% of women with both complaints were scored in classes I, II, III or IV of endometriosis respectively ($p = 0.03$ for infertility versus pain).

Depth of infiltration of endometriosis

In the women with endometriosis maximal depths of infiltration of 1–2,

3–4, 5–6, 7–8, 9–10 and > 10 mm were found in 44, 13, 12, 5, 9 and 8% respectively. The depth of infiltration of pelvic endometriosis ($p < 0.0001$) was significantly higher in women with pelvic pain than in women with infertility alone (Figure 1).

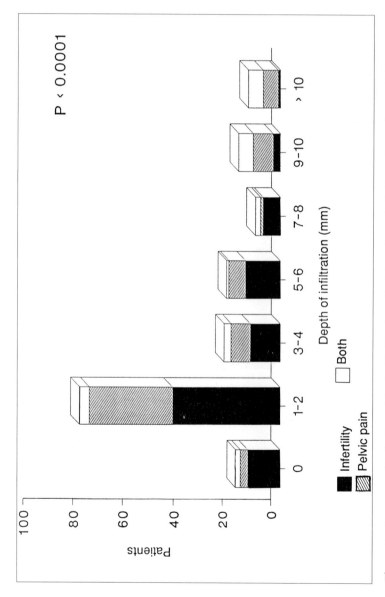

Figure 1 Frequency distribution of depth of infiltration of pelvic endometriosis (0 = endometrioma only) in women with infertility, pelvic pain or both

The depth of infiltration was significantly higher in older women ($p = 0.04$ for lesions deeper than 8 mm). Although the depth of the deepest lesion did not correlate with the age of the woman, the shape of the lesions became more cylindrical and less superficial with increasing age (Table 1).

Table 1   The age of the women and the total volume, peritoneal surface and depth of infiltration of endometriosis. The shape of the endometriotic lesion is obtained by the ratio of the volume up to 1 mm of depth (superficial), up to 4 mm (intermediate) and up to 8 mm (deep) to the total volume. Spearman correlation coefficients, and means ± SD are indicated

Age *(Y)*	n	*Volume* *(cm³)*	*Area* *(cm²)*	*Volume/total volume*		
				Superfic.	*Intermed.*	*Deep*
< 25	31	2.4 ± 3.2	6.7 ± 7.0	.43 ± 25	.87 ± 21	.96 ± 11
26 – 30	67	1.7 ± 2.5	5.1 ± 6.2	.52 ± 32	.25± 23	.93 ± 15
31 – 35	54	1.7 ± 2.7	4.8 ± 8.0	.49 ± 33	.84 ± 23	.93 ± 16
36 – 40	27	2.5 ± 2.8	6.3 ± 7.1	.40 ± 28	.80 ± 26	.91± 18
41 – 45	4	1.7 ± 2.0	2.0 ± 1.5	.23 ± 23	.59 ± 35	.77 ± 22
P		NS	NS	0.16	0.06	0.04

Deeply infiltrating endometriosis in contrast with superficial lesions (Figure 2) was found exclusively in the rectovaginal septum, the uterosacral ligaments and less frequently in the uterovesical fold ($p = 0.002$). Deep endometriosis presented macroscopically (Figure 3) only as gunshot lesions or as white plaques ($p < 0.0001$).

Depth of infiltration and rAFS classification

As could be anticipated, deeply infiltrating pelvic endometriosis is poorly reflected in the rAFS score ($n = 163$, $r = 0.13$, $p = 0.08$) in contrast with the total area of endometriosis ($r = 0.81$, $p = 0.0001$), the presence of endometriomas ($r = 0.66$, $p < 0.0001$), and probably the amount of adhesions present.

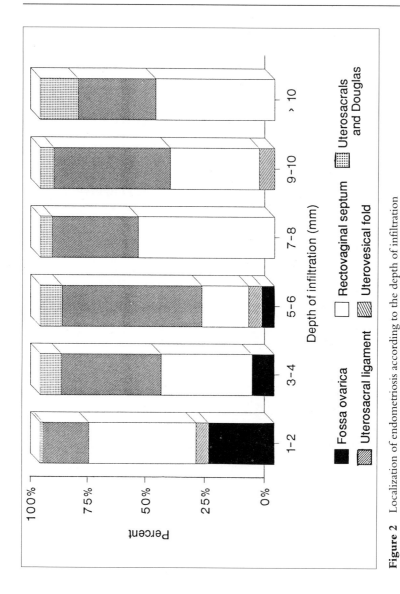

Figure 2 Localization of endometriosis according to the depth of infiltration

CA-125 concentration in plasma and peritoneal fluid

The plasma concentrations correlated with the rAFS classification of endometriosis ($p = 0.0008$, $n = 89$), while the peritoneal fluid concentrations did not (Table 2).

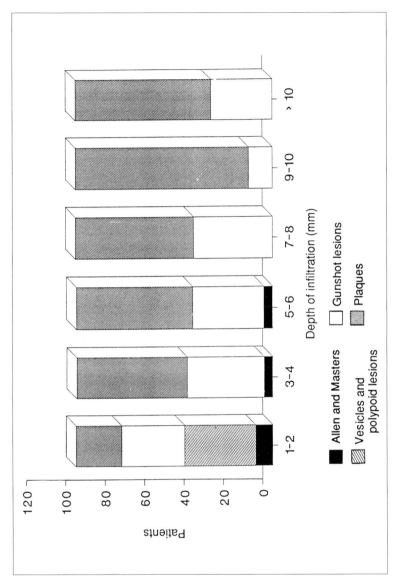

Figure 3 Laparoscopic appearance of pelvic endometriosis according to the depth of infiltration

Table 2 Plasma and peritoneal fluid concentrations of CA-125 in women with endometriosis according to the rAFS classification. The mean ±SD, the Spearman correlation, and the number of samples ( ) are indicated

CA-125 (U/ml)	I	II	III	IV	P
Plasma	18±16 (30)	19±13 (27)	27±14 (17)	62±37 (7)	0.0008
Peritoneal fluid	1328±820 (22)	3889±13610 (27)	1630±1670 (14)	4750±6082 (7)	N.S.

Neither plasma nor peritoneal fluid concentrations correlated with the total area nor the total volume of pelvic endometriosis. The presence of endometriomas, however, strongly correlated with the plasma CA-125 concentration ($p = 0.0004$, $n = 89$), but the volume of the endometriomas did not ($n = 26$).

The shape of the endometriotic lesion predicted both plasma and peritoneal fluid CA-125 concentrations: plasma concentrations were positively correlated, while peritoneal fluid concentrations were negatively correlated with a deep and cylindrical shape (Table 3).

Table 3 Spearman correlations and *P* values ( ) between plasma and peritoneal fluid CA-125 concentrations and the shape of the endometriotic lesion (volume/total volume) up to 1, 3, 4, 8 and 10 mm of depth

CA-125 (U/ml)	n	1	3	4	8	10
Plasma	79	-0.12 (0.29)	-0.21 (0.05)	-0.20 (0.07)	-0.15 (0.18)	0.02 (0.88)
Peritoneal fluid	64	-0.02 (0.85)	0.05 (0.68)	0.13 (0.31)	0.25 (0.04)	0.27 (0.03)

Histopathology of deep infiltrating endometriosis

Light microscopic examination of deep, infiltrating endometriotic lesions revealed several peculiar histological characteristics. Deep infiltration was always arrested at the border of the subperitoneal fibromuscular tissue and the underlying fat tissue. Infiltration into the fibromuscular tissue occurred along the loose connective tissue septa. These septa were completely invaded by ectopic stromal cells embedding small and active glands. Finally, infiltration was sometimes arrested at an intermediate depth of 4–5 mm and, in that case, cystic dilatation of ectopic glands was usually observed. The lining epithelium of these cystic glands had an undifferentiated aspect, lacking any sign of cellular proliferation or secretion.

Cellular activity was observed in 58, 25 and 68% of superficial (< 1mm) intermediate (2–4 mm) and deep lesions respectively and was in phase with the eutopic endometrium in 57, 38 and 74% respectively.

DISCUSSION

The incidence of endometriosis in our study is comparable with that reported in the literature[15]. Also, the frequency distribution of the depth of infiltration is comparable with the recent data of Martin and colleagues[13].

The presence of deep, infiltrating endometriosis has been recognised during hysterectomy for many years. Only the CO_2 laser excision techniques permitted the systematic study of deep pelvic endometriosis in younger women not requiring a hysterectomy. Its relatively frequent occurrence was rather unexpected[13].

Our data strongly suggest that deep pelvic endometriosis should be considered as a separate variety of endometriosis, distinct from superficial (and active), from intermediate (and inactive) endometriosis and from endometriomas. Firstly, deep endometriosis is strongly associated with the occurrence of pelvic pain, almost all women with lesions deeper than 1 cm suffering badly. Secondly, CA-125 concentrations strongly suggest the following mechanism: the release of CA-125 from superficial pelvic endometriosis is directed mainly towards the peritoneal cavity, while deep lesions release their CA-125 mainly into the bloodstream. This hypothesis is appealing, since it is consistent with the finding in superficial and infiltrating carcinomas[16]. Thirdly, and this is the strongest argument, superficial and deep endometriosis are both morphologically very active diseases, while intermediate endometriosis is rather inactive with cystic glandular dilatations[14,17].

The correlation between the rAFS classification and the plasma concentrations of CA-125[18] is mainly due to the strong correlation between plasma CA-125 concentrations and the presence of endometriomas, which contribute strongly to the rAFS classes III and IV.

In order to explain the mechanism of deep infiltration the following hypothesis is suggested. Endometriosis infiltrates progressively deeper and deeper in some women, as can be derived from the association between depth and age of the woman. Infiltration occurs only through the loose connective tissue septa of fibromuscular tissue, as evidenced by its microscopic appearance and by the absence of invasion into fat tissue. This also explains why deep endometriosis is confined uniquely to the pouch of Douglas, the uterosacral ligaments, and the uterovesical fold.

Steroid hormone concentrations are much higher in peritoneal fluid than in plasma, not only in the luteal phase, but also in the follicular phase, where several nanograms of progesterone per ml are found[19,20]. In order to explain the difference in activity between superficial, intermediate and deep pelvic endometriosis, we suggest that superficial endometriosis is probably influenced and inhibited by, possibly, progesterone from peritoneal fluid. Endometriosis at an intermediate depth of infiltration constitutes the phase of inactivation, the so-called burnt out lesions. Once a certain depth of infiltration is obtained however, estimated at 4–5 mm, we suggest that the influence of peritoneal fluid wanes, and endometriosis as a consequence behaves more aggressively, infiltrating more rapidly and inducing pelvic pain.

It is clear that the rAFS classification, which principally is intended to predict fertility outcome after surgery, does not take into account the deep and infiltrating pelvic endometriosis.

The significance of deep pelvic endometriosis for infertility and pain treatment is not yet established. One should be aware, however, that only excisional surgery is able to remove deep endometriosis and to judge depth of infiltration. The continuance of pain relief for many months after medical treatment[20,21], at least in some women, suggests that these drugs act specifically in the case of deep pelvic endometriosis, since they only inactivate superficial endometriosis temporarily[21,22].

In conclusion we described the occurrence, localization and appearance of deeply infiltrating endometriosis as well as its association with pelvic pain. Since deep lesions are active, while intermediate ones are relatively inactive, we postulate a mechanism of infiltration of endometriosis when the inhibitory role of peritoneal fluid diminishes once a depth of 4–5 mm has been reached. From the concentrations of CA-125 in plasma and peritoneal fluid it is concluded that superficial pelvic endometriosis mainly releases CA-125 into the peritoneal cavity, while deep disease (as well as endometriomas) release CA-125 mainly into the bloodstream.

Acknowledgements

Dr S. Demeyere is acknowledged for his invaluable help in the operating theatre and for the collection of data. The morphological evaluation and processing was done in collaboration with Professor Lauweryns (Laboratory of Histopathology). Professor E. Lesaffre (Department of Epidemiology) is thanked for his statistical advice. The assay of CA-125 was done in collaboration with Professor Deroo and Dr De Vos of the Department of Nuclear Medicine. Mrs C. Dewit has taken care of all assays together with Mr M. Gerits, while Mrs M. Verheyden is thanked for the histopathological processing. We are indebted to Mrs M. Mommaerts for typing the manuscript.

REFERENCES

1. Sampson, J.A. (1922). The life history of ovarian hematoma "Hemorrhagic cysts" of endometrial "Mullerian" type. *Am. J. Obstet. Gynecol.*, **4**, 451–512
2. Sampson, J.A. (1927). Peritoneal endometriosis due to the menstrual dissemination of endometrial tissue into the peritoneal cavity. *Am. J. Obstet. Gynecol.*, **14**, 422–9
3. Koninckx, P.R., Ide, P., Vandenbroucke, W. and Brosens, I. (1980). New aspects of the pathophysiology of endometriosis and associated infertility. *J. Reprod. Med.*, **24**, 257–60
4. Dmowski, W.P. (1987). Immunological aspects of endometriosis. *Contr. Gynecol. Obstet.*, **16**, 48–55
5. Halme, J., Becker, S., Hammond, M.G., *et al.* (1983). Increased activation

of pelvic macrophages in infertile women with mild endometriosis. *Am. J. Gynecol.*, **145**, 333–7

6. El-Mahgoub, S. and Yaseen, S. (1980). A positive proof for the theory of coelomic metaplasia. *Am. J. Obstet. Gynecol.*, **137**, 137–40

7. Merrill, J.A. (1966). Endometrial induction of endometriosis across millipore filter. *Am. J. Obstet. Gynecol.*, **94**, 780–90

8. Jansen, R. and Russell, P. (1986). Nonpigmented endometriosis: clinical, laparoscopic and pathologic definition. *Am. J. Obstet. Gynecol.*, **155**, 1154–9

9. Stripling, M., Martin, D., Chatman, D., Vander Zwaag, R. and Poston, W. (1988). Subtle appearance of pelvic endometriosis. *Fertil. Steril.*, **49**, 427–31

10. Vasquez, G., Cornillie, F., and Brosens, I. (1984). Peritoneal endometriosis: scanning electron microscopy and histology of minimal pelvic endometriotic lesions. *Fertil. Steril.*, **42**, 696–703

11. Redwine, D.B. (1987). The distribution of endometriosis in the pelvis by age groups and fertility. *Fertil. Steril.*, **47**, 173–5

12. Martin, D. and Vander Zwaag, R. (1987). Excisional techniques with the CO_2 laser laparoscope. *J. Reprod. Med.*, **32**, 753–8

13. Martin, D., Hubert, G. and Levy, B. (1989). Depth of infiltration of endometriosis. *J. Gynecol. Sur.*, **5**, 55–9

14. Cornillie, F.J., Oosterlynck, D., Lauweryns, J.M. and Koninckx, P.R. (19—). Deeply infiltrating pelvic endometriosis: histology and clinical significance. *Fertil. Steril.* (In press)

15. Martin, D., Hubert, G., Vander Zwaag, R. and El-Zeky, F. (1989). Laparoscopic appearances of peritoneal endometriosis. *Fertil. Steril.*, **51**, 63–7

16. Pavesi, F., Lotzniker, M., Marbello, L., Garbagnoli, P., Franchi, M. and Morattu, R. (1988). CA-125 in benign and malignant diseases involving coelomic epithelium. *J. Tumor Marker Oncol.*, **3**, 49–57

17. Cornillie, F. and Koninckx, P. (1989). Deep, infiltrating pelvic endometriosis: a hitherto undefined disease, different from typical and subtle endometriosis. *2nd World Congress of Endoscopy.* (Clermont-Ferrand) (In press).

18. Barbieri, R.L., Niloff, J.M., Bast, R.C. Jr, Scaetzl, E., Kistner, R.W. and Knapp, R.C. (1986). Elevated serum concentrations of CA-125 in patients with advanced endometriosis. *Fertil. Steril.*, **45**, 630–4

19. Koninckx, P.R., Heyns, W., Verhoeven, G., Van Baelen, H., Lissens, W., and De Moor, P. (1980). Biochemical characterization of peritoneal fluid in women during the menstrual cycle. *J. Clin. Endocrinol. Metabol.*, **51**, 1239–44

20. Donnez, J., Langerock, S. and Thomas, K. (1983). Peritoneal fluid volume, 17β-estradiol and progesterone concentrations in women with endometriosis and/or luteinized unruptured follicle syndrome. *Gynecol. Obstet. Invest.*, **16**, 210–20

21. Evers, J.L. (1988). The second-look laparoscopy for evaluation of the result of medical treatment of endometriosis should not be performed during ovarian suppression. *Fertil. Steril.*, **47**, 502–4

22. Cornillie, F.J., Brosens, I.A., Vasquez, G. and Riphagen, I. (1986). Histological and ultrastructural changes in human endometriotic implants treated with the antiprogesterone steroid ethylnorgestrienone (gestrinone) during two months. *Int. J. Gynecol. Pathol.*, **5**, 95–109

DISCUSSION

Prof. Shaw

Obviously quite wide areas of tissue are excised with laser, including surrounding areas of peritoneum. What is the follow-up of these patients in terms of healing or subsequent adhesion formation with these large raw areas that get left behind?

Prof. Koninckx

The figures are not precisely broken down as between follow-up for fertility and follow-up for pain. In the group of women with pain they are clinically pain free. Up to now I have seen only a few patients with a recurrence of mild pain.

Secondly, as far as fertility is concerned, cumulative pregnancies to date amount to between 60 and 70%. The immediate follow-up is quite astonishing. Although large areas are excised in the pelvis, patients go home the next morning and they go back to work 2 days later.

Dr Cornillie

As a further comment on the direct and immediate follow-up, we usually do a monthly control of the CA-125 levels in the women on whom we have operated, and most of them show a significant decrease of CA-125. At laparoscopy, some patients had values of about 60 units/ml; after surgery values decreased and stayed level in most cases. Most probably these patients who show a significant decrease of CA-125 in plasma had their total volume of endometriosis removed.

Prof. Dr Schweppe

From the clinical point of view the deep invasive endometriosis is endometriosis which reacts to medical therapy only during therapy and recurrences are usually immediate. In the past we have tried to treat these lesions surgically. In this study you have shown active lesions with 80% of them in phase with the cycle. As we know from data of peritoneal superficial endometriosis, endometriosis which is highly differentiated and in phase with the uterine endometrium responds well to medical therapy and recurrences will be quite late. Is there any explanation for these differences?

Prof. Koninckx

I have no answer but I shall try to pass on my thoughts. If we look at the correlation between invasion and pain we know from a number of pieces of published work that the pain will respond very well to treatment with GnRH agonists, and that many of those women remain pain free for a long time after treatment has stopped. I would therefore suggest that GnRH agonists must be doing something special in the deep lesions, and if I was to guess what it is doing, it is making the deep lesions less deep. Once these lesions have a depth of < 4–5mm, they again come under the control of the peritoneal fluid and the woman can remain free of pain for a long time.

4

Clinical and experimental aspects in the medical treatment of endometriosis

M. Dowsett, G. Rose and P. Maouris

INTRODUCTION

Endometriosis is a hormonally responsive disease and its medical treatment is based on the manipulaton of the endocrine environment. The perturbations achieved by some of the agents used vary markedly. We have characterized and compared these changes for danazol, gestrinone and Zoladex which have all been used successfully in the treatment of endometriosis. Since the mechnanism of action of these drugs in relation to endometriosis is not fully understood we examined the effects of these drugs, and some of the endocrine changes which they achieve, on the growth of human endometrial cells *in vitro*. In doing this we followed the principles of investigative pharmacology to distinguish both direct and indirect effects, as illustrated in Figure 1.

ENDOCRINE STUDIES OF DANAZOL, GESTRINONE AND ZOLADEX

Danazol and gestrinone are both steroidal drugs although gestrinone is effective at much lower dosages (at least 100-fold) than danazol. In contrast, Zoladex is a decapeptide, LHRH agonist D–Ser(tBu)^{6}AzaGly^{10} LHRH.

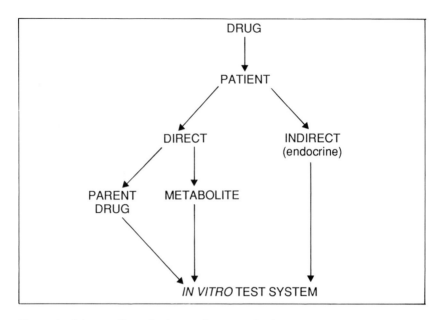

Figure 1 Scheme of investigations to determine the direct and indirect (in this instance endocrine) routes of action of a pharmacological agent

In a study of 20 patients with endometriosis treated with monthly subcutaneous injections of 3.6 mg Zoladex in depot form we found that the compound exerted a profound and predictable ovarian ablation, achieving a steroidal environment consistent with the postmenopausal state. The most apparent change was the reduction in plasma oestrogen levels as a result of reduced gonadotrophin drive. Whilst the mean pretreatment level of oestradiol was 282 ± 40 (SEM) pmol/l (between days 1 and 7 of the menstrual cycle), Figure 2 shows that the distribution of on-treatment values was typically postmenopausal (logarithmically distributed with few values > 100 pmol/l). There were minor falls in the mean levels of testosterone and androstenedione (by about 20 and 15%, respectively). These falls probably reflect a decrease in ovarian androgen synthesis. There was no significant change in the levels of sex hormone-binding globulin (SHBG).

In contrast, in a study of 51 patients who were randomized to treatment with gestrinone (2.5 mg twice weekly) or danazol (200 mg twice daily) we found no significant fall in plasma levels of LH and FSH

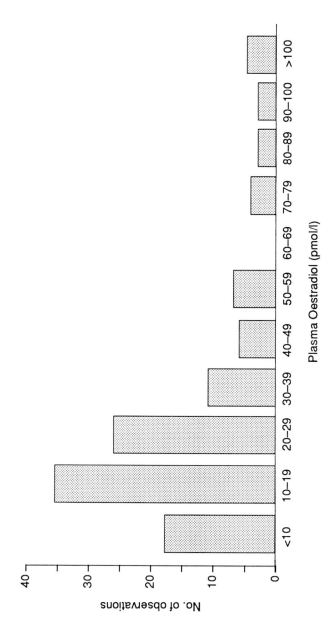

Figure 2 The distribution of 117 plasma oestradiol levels in 20 patients during treatment with monthly subcutaneous injections of 3.6 mg Zoladex for 6 months. Six measurements were made in 19 patients and 3 in the other patient. In each case the measurement was made just prior to the next injection

and only relatively minor changes in oestradiol levels (danazol: Pre [mostly day 15–21] 503 ± 66; month 6, 279 ± 89 pmol/l; gestrinone: Pre, 421 ± 52; month 6, 278 ± 50 pmol/l).

The most marked endocrine change found with these two steroidal agents was a profound fall in SHBG levels. We have demonstrated in a previous study that for danazol this fall is dose related[1]. The significance of this fall relates to the change in the biological activity of testosterone which results. We have shown that for danazol the fall in SHBG levels is associated with a three- to fourfold rise in the proportion of testosterone in the free, biologially active form. However, since there is a concomitant fall in total testosterone concentration, the increase in the *concentration* of free testosterone is between 50 and 100%. The comparative study of gestrinone and danazol demonstrated that gestrinone had quantitatively similar effects on each of these parameters.

The clinical significance of this increase in biologically active testosterone is twofold. Firstly, both of these drugs have androgenic side-effects which may be at least partially due to these endocrine changes. Secondly, since androgens themselves have been found to be effective in the treatment of endometriosis[2] these increases in biologically active testosterone may provide an indirect route by which gestrinone and danazol are pharmacologically active.

INVESTIGATIONS WITH CULTURED HUMAN ENDOMETRIAL CELLS

Having established that the major endocrine effects of Zoladex and the two steroidal drugs were oestrogen deprivation and increased androgenicity, respectively, the effect of these perturbations was examined on the growth of human endometrial cells *in vitro*. The direct effects on growth of danazol and gestrinone were also examined as were the effects of the two major metabolites of danazol, i.e. ethisterone and 2-hydroxymethylethisterone (2OHME).

The technique used for culturing the endometrial cells has been described in detail elsewhere[3]. Briefly, normal human endometrial biopsy samples obtained from the first half of the menstrual cycle were chopped finely, digested enzymatically and placed into monolayer cell culture for 96 hours. The first 24 hours provided a period of pre-incubation after which the medium was changed to introduce test substances. The cells were trypsinized and counted after the 96 hours and the number was compared to that in a non-treated control. All tests were conducted in triplicate. The dosages of the drugs tested were those expected under therapeutic conditions, and for gestrinone, danazol and testosterone 10-fold higher doses were also examined (Table 1).

Table 1 Concentrations of steroids tested for their effect on the growth of endometrial cells in culture. The doses were chosen to be equivalent to the expected circulating levels of the compounds in treated patients (lower dose where 2 are shown). 2OHME = 2 hydroxymethylethisterone

Steroid	*Dose*
Danazol	1×10^{-6}M, 1×10^{-5}M
Ethisterone	2.5×10^{-7}M
2OHME	3×10^{-6}M
Gestrinone	3×10^{-8}, 3×10^{-7}M
Testosterone	2×10^{-9}M, 2×10^{-8}M

The effects found with the steroidal compounds are summarized in Figure 3. Ethisterone, 2OHME and gestrinone had no significant effect on cell growth but both testosterone and danazol caused a marked and highly significant reduction in cell growth which was dose-related.

We were unable to demonstrate any consistent effect of oestradiol on the growth of the cells. This may be because the cells were grown in medium containing a concentration of phenol red (30 µmol/l) which would be expected to have an oestrogenic potency equivalent to approximately 500 pmol oestradiol/l. The effect of added oestrogen would be expected to be much reduced in these circumstances.

CONCLUSIONS

Our data indicate that of the three drugs investigated only danazol has a direct effect on endometrial cell growth *in vitro* and that this is by virtue of the parent drug, and not its metabolites. The endocrine changes

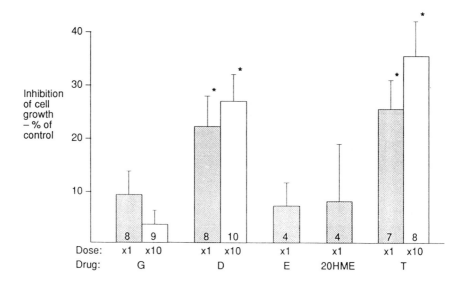

Figure 3 Drug-induced inhibition of the growth of normal endometrial cells in culture. In each case the bar represents the SEM. G, gestrinone; D, danazol; E, ethisterone; 2OHME, 2 hydroxymethylethisterone; T, testosterone. *P < 0.001 versus control. The numbers of patients appear on each bar

achieved by the drugs are profound but markedly different between Zoladex and the steroidal drugs. Oestrogen withdrawal appears to be the key route of pharmacological action for Zoladex, but for gestrinone and danazol oestrogen deprivation *per se* does not appear to be a major mode of action. The observation that testosterone is antiproliferative in our *in vitro* model system indicates that at least part of the pharmacological activity of gestrinone and danazol may be due to the increase in the biological activity of testosterone which they induce.

ACKNOWLEDGEMENTS

We are very grateful to Joanne Nicholls for her excellent technical assistance during this work and to Mr D.K. Edmonds for the supply of biopsy tissue.

REFERENCES

1. Forbes, K.L., Dowsett, M., Rose, G.R., Mudge, J.E. and Jeffcoate, S.L. (1986). Dosage-related effects of danazol on sex hormone-building globulin and free and total androgen levels. *Clin. Endocrinol.*, **25**, 597–605
2. Preston, S.N. and Campbell, H.B. (1953). Pelvic endometriosis. Treatment with methyl testosterone. *Obstet. Gynecol*, **2**, 152–7
3. Rose, G.L., Dowsett, M., Mudge, J.E., White, J. and Jeffcoate, S.L. (1988). The inhibitory effects of danazol, danazol metabolites, gestrinone and testosterone on the growth of human endometrial cells *in vitro*. *Fertil. Steril.*, **49**, 224–8

DISCUSSION

Prof. Seppala

In the data you have presented were you using endometriosis cultures or endometrial cultures?

Dr Dowsett

We did attempt to grow endometriosis in the first instance, but the first pieces of tissue we were obtaining from the surgeons were very fibrotic and the numbers of cells which we were able to obtain in suspension were very small indeed. So unfortunately we had to use normal endometrium and hope that our results were pertinent to endometriotic tissue.

Dr Zullo

I should like to know two details of the cell culture; the concentration of ethanol used in the last culture after 24 hours, and the method of solubilisation of danazol.

Dr Dowsett

The final concentration of ethanol was 0.5% and we added the same amount of ethanol to the control cultures. We found that danazol was sufficiently soluble to obtain those concentrations in ethanol.

5

Receptor mechanisms in endometriotic and endometrial tissue

A. Bergqvist

INTRODUCTION

All hormones mediate their message to the target cells through receptors. For several years the steroid receptors were regarded as localized mainly in the cytoplasm, where they were thought to bind the hormone. The steroid–receptor complex was then transported to the nucleus, where it was bound to the chromatin chain. Thus, initially most studies on steroid receptors were performed in cytosol preparations.

In recent years, our knowledge of this area has changed and today we know that steroid receptors, both in the presence and the absence of steroids, are localized mainly to the nuclei of target cells[1]. The receptors found in the cytosol derive partly from the nuclear compartment and have come into the cytosol after mechanical destruction during preparation. Nuclear receptors appear in two forms, one more loosely bound to the chromatin chain than the other.

In uterine endometrium the oestrogen receptor (ER) level has a maximum in the late proliferative phase, and the progesterone receptor (PR) level has a maximum at ovulation and the early secretory phase.

ASSAY METHODS

The most common methods for steroid receptor assays have been biochemical binding techniques using different types of ligands, usually radioactively labelled synthetic steroids. The one most widely used is the dextran-coated charcoal (DCC) method[2]. Usually the data are plotted according to Scatchard[3] to obtain the quantitative and kinetic characteristics of the binding. Isoelectric focusing in polyacrylamide gel (IFPAG) combined with limited proteolysis is an extensive refinement of the DCC method[4]. Other binding techniques are the sucrose gradient method and the hydroxyl apatite method. Binding techniques only assay receptors unoccupied by endogenous hormones and might also assay some previously occupied receptors after and exchange procedure.

Over the last few years, specific monoclonal antibodies directed towards ER and PR, respectively, have been developed[5]. These antibodies may be used for quantitative assays in tissue homogenates as well as for receptor localization in histological sections. The immunological techniques assay both occupied and unoccupied receptors but give no information whether the receptors assayed are biologically active or not. There is usually a good correlation between biochemical methods and enzyme immunoassays[6].

ENDOMETRIOTIC TISSUE IS USUALLY OESTROGEN DEPENDENT

Endometriosis is found almost exclusively in women in the reproductive age indicating the oestrogen dependence of the tissue. Much less frequently endometriotic lesions are found in postmenopausal women. In such cases these lesions probably existed previously in the fertile period and became reactivated by high endogenous levels of oestrogen associated with obesity or oestrogen replacement therapy. Animal experiments have shown that endometriotic tissue is in most cases dependent on oestrogen for proliferation and for long time survival[7,8]. This oestrogen dependence of endometriotic tissue is the basis for hormonal treatment, leading to ovarian inactivation and oestrogen deprivation of the endometriotic tissue. However, about 20% of endometriotic patients are clinically non-responders to hormonal treatment, which suggests that the endometriotic tissue in these cases is not dependent on the endogenous hormones and not influenced by exogenous hormones. These differences might depend on different steroid receptor levels in the endometriotic lesions.

HISTOLOGY OF ENDOMETRIOTIC TISSUE COMPARED WITH UTERINE ENDOMETRIUM

The histological similarity between endometriotic tissue and uterine endometrium is well known. However, extensive light microscopic and electron microsopic studies of the two tissue types have revealed dissimilarities[9,10]. Endometriotic tissue reacts in a different manner to the endocrine milieu than does endometrium. Endometriotic tissue changes often but not always cyclically according to the hormonal changes during the menstrual cycle. About 20–25% of endometriotic samples show a poor differentiation and do not respond to hormonal influence, indicating an autonomous growth. A complete homogenously performed secretory transformation is uncommon in endometriotic tissue. These findings suggest an incomplete response of endometriotic tissue to the prevalent hormonal milieu depending on a low steroid receptor level.

ER AND PR ASSAYS WITH LIGAND TECHNIQUES

The above data, among others, have focused interest on the cellular receptors for steroid hormones. In the small number of published studies on ER and PR in endometriotic tissue, different ligand techniques have been used (Table 1). The first study on steroid receptors in endometriotic tissue was published in 1979 by Tamaya and colleauges[11]. They studied tissue samples from seven women of whom one was on combined contraceptive pills. In the other six cases ER and PR levels in cytosol (ER_c and PR_c) were measureable in all endometriotic samples. In most of the five cases where ER and PR were assayed also in the endometrium, the receptor levels were lower in the pathological tissue. Since then a few other groups have studied the ER and PR levels in endometriotic tissue. In the study published by the Oulu group in 1980[12], the PR_c level was reported to be high and the ER_c level low in endometriotic tissue. In our first study of 20 women[13] comparing endometriotic tissue and uterine endometrium obtained simultaneously from the same woman, we found

55

Table 1 The number of endometriotic and endometrial samples containing ER and PR in the five studies published where ligand techniques have been used

Author	Number	Endometriotic tissue (n)		Endometrium (n)	
		ER_c+	PR_c+	ER_c+	PR_c+
Tamaya et al. 1979[11]	7*	6/7	6/7	6/6	5/6
Bergqvist et al. 1981[13]	20	8/20	2/9	10/12	8/8
Jänne et al. 1981[14]	47	ca 40%	ca 80%	9/9	9/9
Vierikko et al. 1985[21]	52	38/52	49/52	–	–
Lyndrup et al. 1987[15]	14	9/14	12/12	12/14	13/14

ER = estrogen receptor; PR = progesterone receptor; c = cytosol
* one woman on contraceptive pills

that both ER_c and PR_c were markedly lower in endometriotic tissue than in uterine endometrium. Sometimes the receptors were not even detectable. In the next publication from the Oulu group[14] they added some patients from whom they had obtained uterine endometrium as well. In this study they found a lower PR_c concentration in endometriotic tissue than in endometrium. Also, in the study by Lyndrup and colleagues[15] both ER_c and PR_c were lower in endometriotic tissue than in endometrium.

Thus, the results from all study groups have consistently shown that, at least when biochemical techniques are used, the levels of ER_c and PR_c are markedly lower in endometriotic tissue than in endometrium. The low detection rate with these techniques and the partly contradictory results concerning PR levels in one study[12] might be accounted for by differing detection limits at the different laboratories, on methodological discrepancies and different tissue sampling techniques. However, the high frequency of negative samples was confusing as there are so many indications for the steroid dependence of the tissue. Thus there was a need for more sensitive assays.

ER AND PR ASSAYS WITH IMMUNOLOGICAL TECHNIQUES

Using specific monoclonal antibodies towards ER and PR in an enzyme immunoassay EIA, (Abbott Diagnostica), we found that both types of receptors were measurable in all samples, but the levels were lower in endometriotic tissue than in the uterine endometrium obtained simultaneously from the same woman[16] (Figure 1, Table 2). These results confirm that the ER level is consistently lower in endometriotic tissue than in endometrium. The level of ER_c did not change in endometriotic tissue as pronouncedly as in uterine endometrium during the menstrual cycle. As ER function is regarded as a prerequisite for the synthesis of PR, the PR level indicates biologically active ER in endometriotic tissue. With this method no significant differences in PR_c level between the two tissue types were found. The pronounced discrepancy between PR_c levels found with ligand technique and PR_c levels found with monoclonal antibodies might indicate that the PR assayed with immunological techniques are not always biologically active. The PR level in the nuclear fraction (PR_n) found with EIA is significantly lower

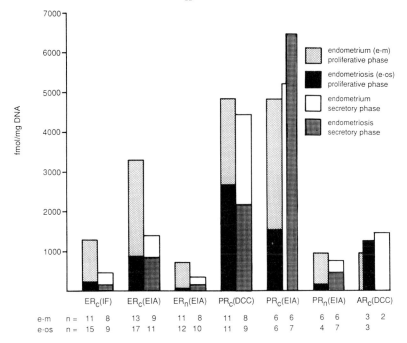

Figure 1 Mean values of ER and PR levels in cytosol (c) and nuclear (n) fraction in endometriotic tissue and endometrium during proliferative and secretory phase studied with ligand techniques and enzyme immunoassays

IF = isoelectric focusing in polyacrylamide gel; EIA = enzyme immunoassay; DCC = dextran coated charcoal method

Table 2 ER, PR and AR levels (mean and standard deviation) in cytosol (c) and nuclear (n) fraction in endometriotic tissue and endometrium assayed with biochemical assays and immunoassays

| | Endometriotic tissue | | Endometrium | |
	n	Mean ± SD	n	Mean ± SD
ER_cIF	25	199 ± 216	20	942 ± 894
ER_cEIA	31	879 ± 1033	24	2464 ± 1774
ER_nEIA	24	179 ± 334	20	555 ± 545
PR_cDCC	21	2355 ± 3011	20	4521 ± 4891
PR_cEIA	15	4116 ± 5515	13	4943 ± 3780
PR_nEIA	13	413 ± 472	13	827 ± 1115
AR_cDCC	4	943 ± 969	5	1136 ± 861

ER = estrogen receptor; PR = progesterone receptor; AR = androgen receptor; c = cytosol; n = nuclei; IF = isoelectric focusing in polyacrylamide gel; EIA = enzyme immunoassay; DCC = dextran coated charcoal method

in endometriotic tissue than in endometrium. The highest level of ER and PR in the menstrual cycle appeared later in endometriotic tissue than in endometrium (Figure 2). These data indicate a different steroid receptor regulation in endometriotic tissue than in endometrium and might explain the sparsity of secretory changes seen histologically in endometriotic tissue.

HISTOCHEMICAL LOCALIZATION OF ER AND PR

The specific monoclonal antibodies may also be used for localization of ER and PR in tissue sections. Three histochemical studies of ER and PR localization have been published comparing endometriotic tissue to uterine endometrium using monoclonal antibodies[17-19]. In all three studies the binding of the specific antibodies was found to be almost exclusively to the nuclei, both in the glandular epithelium and in the stroma in the two tissue types (Figures 3 and 4). Histochemical grading was performed according to percentage of positive cells and intensity of staining. There was a tendency toward stronger binding in endometrium than in

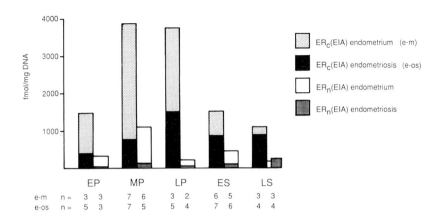

Figure 2 Mean values of ER and PR levels in cytosol (c) and nuclear (n) fractions in endometriotic tissue and endometrium in the different menstrual phases studied with enzyme immunoassay (EIA)

EP = early proliferative; MP = mid proliferative; LP = late proliferative; ES = early secretory; LS = late secretory

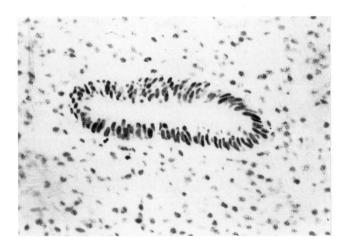

Figure 3 Specific binding of ER to epithelial and stromal cells in endometriotic tissue

endometriotic tissue, but when the two tissue types were in phase there was no obvious difference in binding pattern. There was a marked heterogeneity in the binding pattern in both tissue types.

59

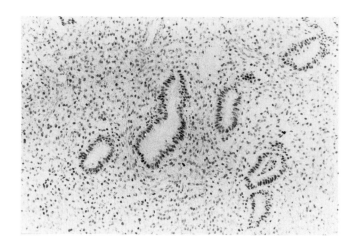

Figure 4   Specific binding of ER to epithelial and stromal cells in endometrium

STEROID RECEPTORS IN THE ENDOMETRIOTIC STROMA

The stroma seems to be of vital importance for the survival of endometriotic glands. A higer PR_C/ER_C ratio has usually been found in endometriotic tissue compared to endometrium[15,18]. As the stromal component in endometriotic tissue usually is smaller than in uterine endometrium, this might indicate that the PR_C level in the stroma is higher in endometriotic tissue than in endometrium.

ANDROGEN RECEPTORS IN ENDOMETRIOTIC TISSUE

Androgen receptors (AR) have been studied in only a few endometriotic samples[11,16,20]. In the few cases where a comparison with uterine endometrium has been carried out, no apparent difference in AR level has been found.

EFFECTS OF EXOGENOUS HORMONES ON STEROID RECEPTOR LEVELS

Under the influence of exogenous hormones such as medroxyprogesterone acetate, danazol and gestrinone, the ER_C and PR_C levels decrease in uterine endometrium[21,22]. However, in endometriotic tissue, neither short- nor long-term treatment induced changes in the receptor levels[23].

OESTROGEN METABOLISM IN ENDOMETRIOTIC TISSUE

Other studies have shown certain differences in the regulation of the oestrogen metabolism in endometriotic tissue compared to that in endometrium[24]. The total hydrolysis of oestrone sulphate (E_1S) as well as the specific formation of oestradiol-17β (E_2) from E_1S was lower in endometriotic tissue than in uterine endometrium, especially in the proliferative phase. E_2 formation and total hydrolysis were correlated in endometriotic tissue but not in endometrium. The 17β-hydroxysteroid oxidoreductase (17β-OHSD) activity, which is responsible for the interconversion between E_2 and oestrone (E_1) is stimulated by progesterone. Vierikko and colleagues[21] found that the activity of this enzyme did not change in endometriotic tissue during the menstrual cycle as it did in endometrium. These results indicate that there are other differences, besides the steroid receptors, in the hormonal regulation of endometriotic tissue and uterine endometrium.

LH RECEPTORS IN ENDOMETRIOTIC TISSUE

Other hormone receptors studied in endometriotic patients are the LH receptors. The LH receptors in ovarian follicles and corpora lutea were lower in endometriotic patients in the early and late follicular phase and in the late luteal phase compared to in control patients. In severe and extensive disease the LH receptor concentration was lower than in mild or moderate endometriosis[25]. One possible explanation for this disturbed LH receptor regulation is the relative hyperprolactinaemia that has been observed in endometriotic patients[26].

DISCUSSION

The collected data on receptor mechanisms in endometriotic tissue concern mainly the steroid receptors. ER, PR and AR are measurable in endometriotic tissue, ER and PR at lower levels than in endometrium and AR in the same range as in normal endometrium. ER are apparently biologically active, but the response to hormonal influence is different compared to that in endometrium. The ER level does not change during the menstrual cycle in as pronounced a manner as in endometrium. This fact indicates a different regulation of the receptor mechanisms.

The studies on PR have shown interesting differences between binding techniques and immunoassays. The monoclonal antibodies detect a similar level of PR in endometriotic tissue compared to endometrium, in tissue homogenates as well as histochemically. On the other side, binding techniques measure lower PR level in endometriotic tissue compared to in endometrium. These findings indicate that there is a high level of biologically inactive PR in endometriotic tissue. As this difference is not found regarding ER and AR, it indicates a different PR regulation in endometriotic tissue. If there is a defect in PR function in endometriotic tissue, it might explain the sometimes weak or absent clinical response of endometriotic tissue to gestagen therapy. Whether the level of biologically active PR is extremely low in endometriotic tissue in the bad responders remains to be studied. There are no indications that the steroid receptor levels differ in endometriotic lesions of different localizations or in primary contra recurrent disease.

An AR level of the same range as in endometrium might explain the apparent effect of androgen hormones on endometriotic tissue. The low LH receptor level in ovarian follicles and corpora lutea might be a factor contributing to infertility associated with endometriosis.

REFERENCES

1. King, W.J. and Greene, G.L. (1984). Monoclonal antibodies localize oestrogen receptor in the nuclei of target cells. *Nature*, **307**, 745–7
2. Korenman, S.G. (1968). Radio–ligand binding assay of specific estrogens using a soluble uterine macromolecule. *J. Clin. Endocrinol. Metab.*, **28**, 127–30

3. Scatchard, D. (1949). The attractions of proteins for small molecules and ions. *Ann. N.Y. Acad. Sci.*, 660–72

4. Gustafsson, J.-Å., Gustafsson, S.A., Nordenskjöld, B., Okret, S., Silfverswärd, C. and Wrange, Ö. (1978). Estradiol receptor analysis in human breast cancer tissue by isoelectric focusing in polyacrylamide gel. *Cancer Res.*, **38**, 4225–8

5. Greene, G.L. and Jensen, E.V. (1982). Monoclonal antibodies as probes for estrogen receptor detection and characterisation. *J. Steroid Biochem.*, **16**, 353–9

6. Fernö, M., Borg, Å. and Sellberg, G. (1986). Enzyme immunoassay of the estrogen receptor in breast cancer biopsy samples. A comparison with isoelectric focusing. *Acta Radiol.*, **25**, 171–5

7. DiZerga, G.S., Barber, D.L. and Hodgen, G.D. (1980). Endometriosis: role of ovarian steroids in initiation, maintenance, and suppression. *Fertil. Steril.*, **33**, 649–53

8. Bergqvist, A., Jeppsson, S., Kullander, S. and Ljungberg, O. (1985). Human uterine endometrium and endometriotic tissue transplanted into nude mice. Morphological effects of various steroid hormones. *Am. J. Pathol.*, **121**, 337–41

9. Schweppe, K.-W., Wynn, R.M. and Beller, F.K. (1984). Ultrastructural comparison of endometriotic implants and eutopic endometrium. *Am. J. Obstet. Gynecol.*, **148**, 1024–39

10. Bergqvist, A., Ljungberg, O. and Myhre, E. (1984). Human endometrium and endometriotic tissue obtained simultaneously: a comparative histological study. *Int. J. Gynecol. Pathol.*, **3**, 135–45

11. Tamaya, T., Motoyama, T., Ohono, Y., Ide, N., Tsurusaki, T. and Okada, H. (1979). Steroid receptor levels and histology of endometriosis and adenomyosis. *Fertil. Steril.*, **31**, 396–400

12. Jänne, O., Kauppila, A., Syrjälä, P. and Vihko, R. (1980). Comparison of cytosol estrogen and progestin receptor status in malignant and benign tumor-like lesions of human ovary. *Int. J. Cancer*, **25**, 175–9

13. Bergqvist, A., Rannevik, G. and Thorell, J. (1981). Estrogen and progesterone cytosol receptor concentrations in endometriotic tissue and intrauterine endometrium. *Acta Obstet. Gynecol. Scand.*, Suppl. **101**, 53–8

14. Jänne, O., Kauppila, A., Kokko, E., Lantto, T., Rönnberg, L. and Vihko, R. (1981). Estrogen and progestin receptors in endometriosis lesions: comparison with endometrial tissue. *Am. J. Obstet. Gynecol.*, **141**, 562–6

15. Lyndrup, J., Thorpe, S., Glenthøj, A., Obel, E. and Sele, V. (1987). Altered progesterone/estrogen receptor ratios in endometriosis. *Acta Obstet. Gynecol. Scand.*, **66**, 625–9

16. Bergqvist, A. and Fernö, M. (1988). Steroid receptors in endometriotic

tissue and endometrium assayed with monoclonal antibodies. In Genazzani, A.R., Petraglia, F., Volpe, A. and Facchinetti, F. (eds). *Recent Research on Gynecological Endocrinology*, **1**, 394-9. (Carnforth, Park Ridge: The Parthenon Publishing Group)

17. Bur, M.E., Greene, G.L. and Press, M.F. (1987). Estrogen receptor localization in formalin-fixed, paraffin-embedded endometrium and endometriotic tissues. *Int. J. Gynecol. Pathol.*, **6**, 140–51

18. Lessey, B.A., Metzger, D.A., Haney, A.F. and McCarty, K.S. Jr. (1989). Immunohistochemical analysis of estrogen and progesterone receptors in endometriosis: comparison with normal endometrium during the menstrual cycle and the effect of medical therapy. *Fertil. Steril.*, **51**, 409–15

19. Bergqvist, A., Ljungberg, O. and Fernö, M. (1989). Histochemical localization of estrogen (ER) and progesterone (PR) receptors in endometriotic tissue and endometrium using monoclonal antibodies. In *The 2nd International Symposium on Endometriosis*, pp.43. (Houston, Texas)

20. Punnonen, R., Pettersson, K., Vanharanta, R. and Lukola, A. (1985). Androgen, estrogen and progestin binding in cytosols of benign gynecologic tumors and tumor-like lesions. *Horm. Metabol. Res.*, **17**, 607–9

21. Vierikko, P., Kauppila, A., Rönnberg, L. and Vihko, R. (1985). Steroidal regulation of endometriosis tissue: lack of induction of 17β-hydroxysteroid dehydrogenase activity by progesterone, medroxyprogesterone acetate, or danazol. *Fertil. Steril.*, **43**, 218–24

22. Tamaya, T. and Okada, H. (1987). Receptors – rationales of steroid therapy for pelvic endometriosis. *Contr. Gynec. Obstet.*, **16**, 170–5

23. Kauppila, A., Rajaniemi, H., Rönnberg, L. and Vihko, R. (1987). Receptor disorders in endometriosis. *Contr. Gynec. Obstet.*, **16**, 40–7

24. Carlström, K., Bergqvist, A. and Ljungberg, O. (1988). Metabolism of estrone sulfate in endometriotic tissue and in uterine endometrium in proliferative and secretory cycle phase. *Fertil. Steril.*, **49**, 229–33

25. Rönnberg, L., Kauppila, A. and Rajaniemi, H. (1984). Luteinizing hormone receptor disorder in endometriosis. *Fertil. Steril.*, **42**, 64–8

26. Acién, P., Lloret, M. and Graells, M. (1989). Prolactin and its response to the luteinizing hormone-releasing hormone thyrotrophin-releasing hormone test in patients with endometriosis before, during, and after treatment with danazol. *Fertil. Steril.*, **51**, 774–80

DISCUSSION

Prof. Shaw

Dr Bergqvist has tried to address what is obviously a very difficult problem and perhaps begs the whole question of whether the endometriotic tissue in its origins is really in common with the endometrium or whether it is actually tissue that is differentiating from other origins and therefore would be expected to have different receptor patterns and responses.

Dr Malinak
Were the histochemical determinations made on fresh or on fixed tissue?

Dr Bergqvist
Fixed and fresh-frozen tissue were compared and the results were much better in the fresh-frozen tissue which we used thereafter.

6

Current medical therapies for endometriosis: a review

K.-W. Schweppe

INTRODUCTION

Endometriosis accounts for 10–20% of all female infertility. Although the disease has been studied for decades, the hormonal requirements for its initiation and maintenance are not fully understood. It is known that hormones secreted by the ovaries are needed for the establishment or continued presence of endometriosis because the disorder occurs only after the onset of puberty and normally disappears after the menopause. Oestrogen supports the growth of ectopic endometrial tissue.

Much effort in basic research has been expended for the better understanding of the hormonal requirements of endometriosis, because knowledge of such requirements might yield clues to treatment. A study by the National Institute of Child Health and Human Development (Pregnancy Research branch)[1] involved implantation of endometrial tissue in the peritoneal cavity of castrated monkeys. By 12 weeks, the endometrial tissue in the control monkeys was no longer viable. The tissue in the groups receiving oestradiol or progesterone or both continued to grow throughout the 16-week study, indicating a requirement for ovarian steroid hormones to maintain endometriotic tissue viability.

THERAPEUTIC STRATEGIES

The treatment of endometriosis is governed mainly by the patients' reproductive expectations. Next in importance are the severity of the symptoms and signs, and the patients' age. The treatment has to be tailored to the individual situation, because no method of treatment will with certainty cure all patients. One of the main reasons for this is the broad morphological variation of endometriosis[2,3]. These authors interpreted the variable degrees of differentiation as indicating immaturity, i.e. as earlier stages on their way of linear differentiation from stem cells to endometrium-like tissue. Systematic ultramorphological analysis reveals the following degrees of differentiation in endometriotic lesions:

(1)   dystrophic variation,

(2)   dissociation of glandular and stromal tissue,

(3)   autonomous modulation with partial endocrine reactivity,

(4)   progressive, polymorphic differentiation.

These variations exist as singular, segmental, mixed or homogenous areas within an endometriotic lesion. In interpreting morphological findings in endometriosis three aspects have to be considered.

(1)   Variable degree of differentiation according to morphological ageing.

(2)   Variable differentiation according to disontogenetic development (genetic mutation).

(3)   Variable degrees of dysplasia.

These three components will decide whether or not endometriosis can be modulated by hormones, i.e. whether hormonal therapeutic regimens will be effective[4]. Up to 70% of patients on hormonal treatment can be expected to experience remission of endometriosis. When assessing the benefits of hormone medication besides pregnancy rates and/or cure of symptoms it is also necessary to consider improvement in the physical signs. Laparoscopy and histological verification performed before and after treatment are needed to prove this point.

Testosterone regimen

About 40 years ago, testosterone and methyltestosterone were introduced for the treatment of endometriosis. Although the mechanism of action of testosterone still remains obscure, many investigators reported on the relief of subjective symptoms such as pelvic pain, dyspareunia and dysmenorrhoea[4]. Methyltestosterone, 5–10 mg daily orally, over a period of 6 months did not sufficiently suppress ovarian function since ovulations and pregnancies were observed during treatment. Alleviation of symptoms was reported in 80% of the cases, but pregnancy rates varied from 11–16%. Serious androgenic side-effects such as hirsutism, acne, deepening of the voice and clitoromegaly were observed in between 5 and 20% of the cases.

Because of these severe side-effects and adverse influences on liver metabolism, androgen therapy today has no place in the treatment of endometriosis.

The five therapeutic principles for medical treatment of endometriosis which have been used during the past three decades are characterized in Table 1.

Table 1 Endocrine effects of medical treatment of endometriosis

	LH	FSH	E2	P	A	Comments
Pseudopregnancy regimen	=	=	‡	‡	nc	decidualisation of endometrium
Progestin only regimen	–	–	–	‡	nc	synthetic C-19 progestins have androgen effects
Danazol	nc	nc	–	–	(+)	inhibition of ovarian steroidogenesis
Gestrinone	–	–	–	–	+	antiprogestational and androgenic effects
GnRH agonists	nc	nc	–	–	–	desensitization of pituitary gland gonadotrophins

nc = no change

Pseudopregnancy regimen

This concept was based on clinical observations of a regression of endometriosis in the last trimester of pregnancy. Kistner[5] reported favourably on pseudocyesis treatment using different oestrogen–progestagen preparations in high dosage. According to our introductory remarks, it is difficult to understand why these treatments should benefit endometriosis.

As for the treatment of pseudopregnancy by high oestrogen medication, this is not undertaken nowadays because of the severe side-effects, both metabolic and systemic, known to ensue.

Progestin-only regimen

Oral progestins without the oestrogen component have also been described as effective in the treatment of endometriosis (Table 2). The hypo-oestrogenic, hypergestagenic status causes decidual transformation of the eutopic endometrium and to some degree in the ectopic lesions too. Theoretically this mode of treatment offers the advantage of improved individual tolerance and lesser oestrogenic side-effects. To induce decidual transformation, however, with resultant necrosis and resorption of the implant, concomitant oestrogen action is required[6]. As continuous progestin therapy results in low serum oestradiol levels, breakthrough bleeding is a common event. Results in general do not vary

Table 2   Clinical results of progesterone treatment

Author	Medication	Cure Rate Laparoscopy	Pregnancy Rate (%)	Recurrence Rate (%)
Korte[23] (1970)	Lynoestrenol	68%★	nr	34%
Johnston[24] (1976)	Dydrogestrone	94%	52%	53%
Moghissi[25] (1976)	Medroxyprogesterone acetate	100%★	46%	9%
Willemsen[26] (1985)	Medroxyprogesterone acetate	50%	nr	nr

★by gynaecological examination only. nr = not reported

greatly from oestrogen–progestin combination therapy. An overview of recurrence rates following progestin therapy is presented in Table 3.

Pregnancy rates following medroxyprogesterone acetate, lynoestrenol or norethisterone acetate regimens vary from 5 to 90% depending on the stage of an endometriosis and whether they were corrected or not. Poor cycle control and early recurrence are major disadvantages of gestagen-only therapy.

A significant drawback to the use of progestin alone is the occasionally prolonged interval to resumption of ovulatory menses after discontinuation. Inadequate data are available regarding the need for surgery subsequent to progestin therapy.

Table 3 Recurrences after progesterone treatment

Author	Medication	Dose mg/d	Duration (months)	Patients n	Recurrences n	(%)
Nevinnystickel[27] (1962)	Norethisterone acetate	10–30	9–12	19	3	16
Hugentobler[28] (1971)	Norethisterone acetate	30	9	18	4	22
Korte et al.[23] (1970)	Lynoestrenol	5	nr	44	15	34
Richter et al.[29] (1981)	Lynoestrenol	5	9	67	8	12
Schindler[30] (1984)	Norethisterone acetate	10–20	6–10	11	3	27

nr = not reported

Danazol regimens

Danazol is an isoxazol derivative of 17α-ethinyltestosterone and its beneficial effects are demonstrated in various other diseases such as benign breast disease, unexplained infertility, precocious puberty, angioneurotic oedema and menorrhagia. Its mechanisms of action are still unclear. Dmowski and Cohen showed the central effects on the hypothalamic–pituitary–ovarian axis[7]. Other authors have suggested a directly suppressive effect through peripheral actions on the target organs[8-10]. Moderate binding of danazol to testosterone, progesterone and glucocorticoid receptors has been shown, but the results regarding progestational, antiprogestational and glucocorticoid properties in man are contradictory[11,12]. Danazol has, however, been shown to be effective in cases of endometriosis and associated infertility (Table 4). Side-effects of danazol include weight gain and sometimes, and more worryingly, androgenic side-effects (Figure 1). These occur in 4 to 23% of the cases treated[4]. On the other hand, there are reports that women taking this drug have normal to low serum testosterone concentrations, which is consistent with a suppressive effect of danazol on ovarian function[13]. Intrinsic androgenicity of danazol then is responsible for major side-effects ranging from anabolic weight gain and muscle cramps to minimal hirsutism and acne. These symptoms are significant but rarely cause the patient to discontinue her medication for these reasons alone.

Apparently, danazol interferes with pulsatile gonadotrophin secretion, has some androgenicity via its main metabolite ethisterone and, despite its low affinity to oestradiol and progesterone receptors, blocks progesterone

Table 4 Clinical results of danazol treatment

Author	Danazol mg/day	Cure Rate % Subj	Cure Rate % Obj	Pregnancy Rate % Gr	Pregnancy Rate % Corr	Recurrence Rate %
Friedlander[31] (1976)	600–800	86	73★	76	nr	nr
Dmowski and Cohen[7] (1978)	800	100	85	46	72	39
Greenblatt and Tzingounis[32] (1979)	800	100	84	33	50	33
Barberi et al.[33] (1982)	800	89	94★	46	nr	33
Buttram et al.[34] (1985)	400–800	nr	51	53	nr	nr
Audebert et al.[35] (1980)	400–800	89	70	50	nr	14
Schweppe[36] (1987)	600	88	69	19	62	35

★by gynaecological examination only. nr = not reported

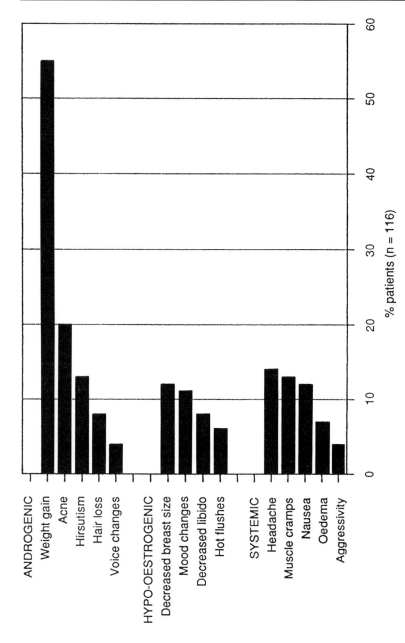

Figure 1 Side-effects during danazol treatment. Six months therapy at 600 mg/day[36]

action at the endometrium, suppressing sex hormone-binding globulin (SHBG) and corticosteriod-binding globulin (CBG) levels and thereby varies binding of testosterone, oestradiol, progesterone and cortisone. Follicle maturation is suppressed and inhibition of the midcycle gonadotrophin surge can be observed[14].

In a recent study, Rönnberg and Järvinen presented a prospective comparative trial of surgical and/or pharmacological therapy in 211 infertile patients with endometriosis[15]. Following 6 months of danazol therapy, the uncorrected pregnancy rate was highest (56%) and the interval between discontinuation of therapy and conception shortest as compared to all other regimens. These authors therefore recommended treatment of endometriosis primarily with danazol, 600 mg for 6 months. In patients with more advanced stages of endometriosis, conservative surgery and postsurgical danazol treatment still achieves a 32% pregnancy rate. In evaluating the distribution of stages (AFS classifications) in this study, patients appear to have been selected to the various treatment regimens. This experience suggested that different modes of treatment have their specific indications with respect to the stage of endometriosis. In the more advanced cases of endometriosis, the more likely it is that a surgical approach is indicated.

With respect to histological differentiation, only those lesions resembling corporal endometrium will have a chance of regression following danazol treatment. Less differentiated endometriosis and mixed forms with tendencies of autonomous proliferation will at best be arrested. Following danazol treatment, one has to be aware of the at least one in three chance of persisting endometriosis.

If danazol treatment is assessed with respect to the results in different stages of endometriosis, it appears that recurrence rates account for 15–20% within the first year following treatment and another 5% for each following year of observation. Henriques and colleagues point out, that according to their findings they expect 50% recurrence 5 years after danazol treatment[16].

Gestrinone therapy

Gestrinone (13-ethyl-17α-ethinyl-17-hydroxy-gona-4,9,11-trien-3-one) is a synthetic trienic 19-nor-steroid with antigonadotrophic properties, which has been used experimentally as a long-acting contraceptive[17]. The effects of gestrinone on the endometrium, include a decrease in oestrogen and progestagen receptors , and induction of 17β-HSD which are characteristic of progestin action[18]. These parameters remained unchanged in endometriotic tissue. The data indicate that gestrinone has effects that are typical of androgens and progestagens.

According to German experiences, side-effects ranged from 22–50%. Follow up 2 years after treatment indicated 8–16% recurrence of symptoms, 45–64% of intrauterine pregnancies and 40–60% living babies. In more than 50% of these patients, the doses had to be increased because of metrorrhagia and spotting as well as continuing menstrual bleeding. However, all of these patients before entering gestrinone therapy, were subjected to thermocoagulation of endometiotic foci visualized during laparoscopic diagnostic procedure. It is within this context that some authors recommend endocoagulation of endometriosis lesions including adhesiolysis, salpingolysis, ovariolysis and fimbrioplasty during diagnostic work up. This is to be followed by a conservative endocrine treatment over a period of at least 6 months with lynoestrenol, danazol and gestrinone and finally, a "second-look" laparoscopy is done, which includes final tubal correction and repeated endocoagulation if necessary (three-step-therapy, Mettler and Semm[19]).

LHRH AGONISTS AND ENDOMETRIOSIS

Since the specific action of LHRH agonists is to reduce or suppress FSH- and LH-secretion, follicular maturation may be arrested via a reversible pituitary blockage of FSH-release. This is the therapeutic principle of antigonadotrophic action of LHRH agonists such as buserelin, narfarelin, or Zoladex. According to a recent review of Sandow[20], the regimens may differ in doses and in mode of administration, depending on the rapidity and level of pituitary suppression.

An important observation is the vast difference in individual dose requirements[21]. Buserelin nasal spray (800–1200 mcg per day for 4–6 months) provided relief of pain in 27/27 patients, and endometrial atrophy was confirmed in 15 patients. In the post-treatment control period, 22 out of 27 patients showed at 6–26 months follow-up laparoscopy formation of scars or at laparotomy fibrosis and atrophy of the endometriotic lesions. The beneficial clinical results were relief of dysmenorrhoea, cessation of bowel bleeding, and three pregnancies in 22 patients treated with the objective of restoring fertility. However, already during this follow-up interval, four recurrences were observed indicating that the treatment provided only temporary suppression of the disease, as is the case with other hormonal approaches to endometriosis. Up to now there have been some clinical trials published about the effectivity of GnRH analogues (Table 5). Our own experience[22] in 52 patients, AFS Stages I–IV, 6 months on 900 mcg buserelin intranasally, since 1984 resulted in a preliminary pregnancy rate of 35%, a regression of endometriosis judged by repeat laparoscopy of 69%, and complete relief of symptoms in 85%. No pathological changes of metabolic pathways have been found and the side-effects (Figure 2) are related to the therapeutic goal – that of inducing hypo-oestrogenism. An unsolved question is the risk

Table 5 Clinical results of GnRH analogues in the treatment of endometriosis

Author	No. of patients	Improvement %		Pregnancy Rate %		Recurrence Rate %
		Subj.	Obj.+	Gr.	Corr	
Lemay et al.[37] (1986)	24	75	48	45	nr	nr
Cirkel et al.[38] (1986)	40	89	50	23	33	nr
Franssen et al.[39] (1986)	23	80	43	26	nr	nr
Cirkel et al.[40] (1989)	64	92	73	38	nr	9.4*
Fuchs et al.[41] (1989)	31	90	87	31	nr	6.5*
Koch et al.[42] (1989)	21	90	65	46	75	10.0*
Bühler et al.[43] (1989)	107	70	44	nr	nr	nr
Schweppe et al.[22] (1989)	52	85	69	35	41	11.4**

+ = reduction of endometriosis in % at control laparoscopy.

★ = follow-up period of 6 months. ★★ = follow-up period of 12 months

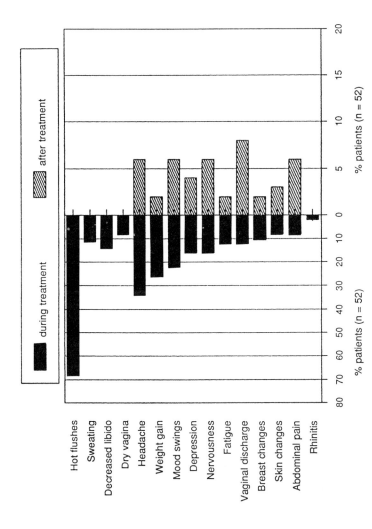

Figure 2 Side–effects during GnRH analogues in the treatment of endometriosis[22]

of induction of osteoporosis. Preliminary data demonstrate a reversible bone loss of 3–5% during a 6 months period of treatment (See later chapters).

CONCLUSION

Gestagens have been widely used in the past, but the mechanisms of action are poorly understood and further basic research is needed. Randomized comparative clinical trials have yet to confirm the impression of beneficial effects on endometriosis-induced subjective complaints. Today the established standard regimen for all stages of endometriosis is danazol – alone or in combination with surgical procedures by pelviscopy or microsurgery. Side-effects – especially androgenic symptoms are frequent, including changes of lipids and liver metabolism. The development of GnRH analogues offers a new therapeutic principle which is effective in relief of symptoms and regression of endometriotic implants. The profile and frequency of side-effects may be the most important difference in comparision with the standard regimens of the past.

REFERENCES

1. DiZerega, G.S., Barber, D.L. and Hodgen, G.D. (1980). Endometriosis: role of ovarian steroids in initiation, maintenance, and suppression. *Fertil. Steril.*, **33**, 649–53
2. Novak, E. and De Lima, O.A. (1948). A correlative study of adenomyosis and pelvic endometriosis, with special reference to the hormonal reaction of ectopic endometrium. *Am. J. Obstet. Gynecol.*, **56**, 634–44
3. Novak, E. and Hoge, A.F. (1958). Endometriosis of the lower genital tract. *Obstet. Gynecol.*, **12**, 687–93
4. Schweppe, K.-W. (1984). *Morphologie und Klinik der Endometriose,* pp. 198–221. (Stuttgart, New York: Schattauer)
5. Kistner, R.W. (1958). The use of newer progestins in the treatment of endometriosis. *Am. J. Obstet. Gynecol.*, **75**, 264–78
6. Hammond, C.B. and Haney, A.F. (1978). Conservative treatment of endometriosis. *Fertil. Steril.*, **30**, 497–509
7. Dmowski, W.P. and Cohen, M.R. (1978). Antigonadotropin (danazol) in

the treatment of endometriosis. *Am. J. Obstet. Gynecol.*, **130**, 41–8

8. Wentz, A.C., Jones, G.S., Sapp, K.C. and King, T.M. (1976). Progestational activity of danazol in the human female subject. *Am. J. Obstet. Gynecol.*, **126**, 378–84

9. Tsang, B.K., Henderson, K.M. and Armstrong, D.T. (1979). Effect of danazol on estradiol and progesterone secretion by porcine ovarian cells *in vitro*. *Am. J. Obstet. Gynecol.*, **133**, 256–9

10. Asch, R.H., Fernandez, E.O., Siler-Khodr, T.M., Bartke, A., and Pauerstein, C.J. (1980). Mechanism of induction of luteal phase defects by danazol. *Am. J. Obstet. Gynecol.*, **136**, 932–40

11. Barbieri, R.L., Lee, H. and Ryan, K.J. (1979). Danazol binding to rat androgen, glucocorticoid, progesterone, and estrogen receptors. *Fertil. Steril.*, **31**, 182–6

12. Dmowski, W.P. (1979). Endocrine properties and clinical application of danazol. *Fertil. Steril.*, **31**, 237–51

13. Sharp, A.M., Fraser, I.S. and Carterson, I.D. (1983). Further studies on danazol interference in testosterone radioimmono assays. *Clin. Chem.*, **29**, 141–3

14. Barbieri, R.L. and Ryan, K.J. (1981). Danazol: endocrine pharmacology and therapeutic applications. *Am. J. Obstet. Gynecol.*, **141**, 453–63

15. Rönnberg, L. and Järvinen, P.A. (1984). Pregnancy rates following various therapy modes for endometriosis in infertile patients. *Acta Obstet. Gynecol. Scand.*, **124**, Suppl., 69–72

16. Henriques, E.S., Jofe, M.H., Friedlander, R.L. and Swarzt, D.P. (1982). Longterm follow up of endometriosis treated with danazol. In Semm, K., Greenblatt, R.B. and Mettler, L. (eds). *Genital Endometriosis and Infertility*. pp. 55–66. (Stuttgart: Thieme)

17. Cotinho, E.M. (1978). Clinical experience with implant contraception. *Contraception*, **18**, 411–17

18. Kauppila, A., Isomaa, U., Rönnberg, L., Vierikko, P. and Vihko, R. (1985). Effects of gestrinone in endometriosis tissue and endometrium. *Fertil. Steril.*, **44**, 466–70

19. Mettler, L. and Semm, K. (1984). Three-step-therapy of genital endometriosis. In Reno, J.P. *et al.* (eds). *Medical Managment of Endometriosis.* pp. 233–47. (New York: Raven)

20. Sandow, J. (1989) Physiologische und pharmakologische Unterngen von Buserelin: Präklinische Untersuchungen. In Schind, A. E. and Schweppe, K.-W. (eds). *Endometriose – neue Therapiemoglichen durch Buserelin.* pp. 23–42. (Berlin: de Gruyter)

21. Schmidt-Gollwitzer, M., Hardt, W. and Borgmann, V. (1985). Antigonadal properties of LH-RH agonists: Therapeutic applications in

human. In Schmidt-Gollwitzer, M. (ed). *LH-RH and its Analogues*. pp. 269–82. (Berlin: de Gruyter)

22. Schweppe, K.-W. and Cirkel, U. (1988). Gn-RH analogues in the treatment of endometriosis: effectivity and side-effects. In *4th Annual Meeting ESHRE*. (Barcelona)

23. Korte, W., Beck, K.J. and Scherholz, K.P. (1970). Operative Behandlung der Endometriose und Langzeittherapie mit Lynestrenol. *Geburtsh. u. Frauenheilk.*, **30**, 122

24. Johnston, W.I.H. (1976). Dydrogesterone and endometriosis. *Br. J. Obstet. Gynaecol.*, **83**, 77

25. Moghissi, K.S. and Boyce, C.R. (1976). Management of endometriosis with oral medroxyprogesterone acetate. *Obstet. Gynecol.*, **47**, 265

26. Willemsen, W.N.P., Rolland. R., Vemer, H.M. and Thomas, C.M.G. (1985). Low versus high medroxyprogesterone acetate in the treatment of endometriosis. *Arch. Gynecol.*, **237**, suppl. abstract 12.79.02

27. Nevinny-Stickel, J. (1962). Die Bedeutung des Gestageneffekts auf das Endometrium für die Behandlung der Endometriose. *Geburtsh. u. Frauenheilk.*, **22**, 689

28. Hugentobler, R. (1971). Die Behandlung der Endometriose mit hochdosiertem Primolut-Nor. *Thesis* (Zürich)

29. Richter, K., Schmidt-Tannwald, I. and Terruhn, V. (1981). Endometriosis externa. 459 histologisch verifizierte Beobachtungen. *Gynäkol. Praxis*, **5**, 97–107

30. Schindler, A.E. (1984). Prognose der Endometriose nach Therapie. *Endometriose*, **3**, 8–12

31. Friedlander, R.L. (1976). Experiences with danazol in therapy of endometriosis. In Greenblatt, R.B. (ed). *Recent Advances in Endometriosis*, p. 100. (Princeton: Exerpta Medica)

32. Greenblatt, R.B. and Tzingounis, V. (1979). Danazol treatment of endometriosis: long term follow-up. *Fertil. Steril.*, **32**, 518

33. Barbieri, R.L., Evans, S. and Kistner, R.W. (1982). Danazol in the treatment of endometriosis: analysis of 100 cases with 4 years follow-up. *Fertil. Steril.*, **37**, 737

34. Buttram, V.C., Reiter, R.C. and Ward, S. (1985). Treatment of endometriosis with danazol. Report of a 6 year prospective study. *Fertil. Steril.*, **43**, 353

35. Audebert, A.J.M., Larue-Charlus, S. and Emperaire, J.C. (1980). Endometriose, infertilité: resultats à moyen terme de 62 cas traités par danazol. *Gynecologie*, **31**, 397

36. Schweppe, K.-W. (1987). Therapieerfolge und Rezidivrate nach Endometriosebehandlung mit danazol. *Endometriose*, **5**, 4–12

37. Lemay, A., Malheux, R., Jean, C. and Faure, N. (1986). Efficacy of different modalities of LHRH agonist (buserelin) administration on the inhibition of pituitary-ovarian axis for the treatment of endometriosis. In Rolland, R., Chadha, D. R. and Willemsen, W.N.P. (eds). *Gonadotrophin Down-regulation in Gynecological Practice*, p. 157. (New York: Alan Liss)

38. Cirkel, U., Schweppe, K.-W., Ochs, H. and Schneider, H.P.G. (1986). Effects of LHRH agonist therapy in the treatment of endometriosis. In Rolland, R., Chadha, D.R. and Willemsen, W.N.P. (eds). *Gonadotrophin Down-regulation in Gynecological Practice*, p. 189. (New York: Alan Liss)

39. Franssen, A.M.H.W., Kauer, F.M., Rolland, R. *et al.* (1986). The effect of agonist therapy in the treatment of endometriosis. In Rolland, R., Chadha, D.R. and Willemsen, W.N.P. (eds). *Gonadotrophin Down-regulation in Gynecological Practice*, p. 201. (New York: Alan Liss)

40. Cirkel, U., Schweppe, K.-W., Ochs, H. and Schneider, H.P.G. (1989). Behandlung der Endometriosis genitalis externa mit Buserelin. In Schinddler, A.E. and Schweppe, K.-W. (eds). *Endometriose – Neue Therapiemöglichkeiten durch Buserelin*, p. 75. (Berlin, New York: W. de Gruyter)

41. Fuchs, U., Zwirner, M. and Keller, E. (1989). Wirkung und Akzeptanz der Buserelintherapie bei Endometriose. In Schinddler, A.E. and Schweppe, K.-W. (eds). *Endometriose – Neue Therapiemöglichkeiten durch Buserelin*, p. 101. (Berlin, New York: W. de Gruyter)

42. Koch, R. (1989). Ergebnisse der Behandlung der Endometriose mit dem GnRH-Analogon Buserelin. In Schinddler, A.E., Schweppe, K.-W. (eds). *Endometriose – Neue Therapiemöglichkeiten durch Buserelin*, p. 111. (Berlin, New York: W. de Gruyter)

43. Bühler, K., Fischer, P., *et al.* (1989). Endometriosetherapie mit Buserelin bei 107 Frauen. In Schinddler, A.E. and Schweppe, K.-W. (eds). *Endometriose – Neue Therapiemöglichkeiten durch Buserelin*, p. 91. (Berlin, New York: W. de Gruyter)

DISCUSSION

Dr Evers
Focusing on danazol, all studies reporting pregnancy results nowadays use the success rate of danazol treatment as the golden standard. I agree that this is correct when judging symptom relief, but with respect to pregnancy figures it is a dangerous habit.

Is there any study in the literature which proves, in a randomized controlled fashion against placebo, that danazol does anything for infertility in an endometriosis patient?

Prof. Schweppe

There is no study with these criteria for any medical treatment of endometriosis. The problem is that in the past treatment studies have primarily been done in a non-randomized way or with selected groups. An unselected prospective comparative trial using these criteria and life tables analysis to judge pregnancy coupled with a prior complete infertility check applying standard criteria has not been done.

Dr Bayot

Is one possible explanation the effectiveness of danazol against antibodies in the endometrium? Such a decrease in antibodies would seem to have been proved. I am not suggesting that other therapies do not have similar effects but it may be that for danazol it is proven.

Prof. Schweppe

Published studies have shown that special antibodies against autologous endometrium decrease in the course of danazol therapy and the levels stay low in the follow-up period of between 6 and 12 months. Other medications such as progesterone or GnRH analogues do not have this effect.

Prof. Koninckx

One of the problems with hormone treatment of endometriosis as regards follow-up of pregnancy is that we are looking at several different types of endometriosis which are all mixed together in the group – superficial, infiltrating and endometriomas. This is one of the main difficulties.

The second difficulty is that duration of infertility is rarely taken into account. Of those who will conceive, between 60 and 70% are pregnant within 2 months, a pregnancy rate of something like 40 to 50% in the first month. Among those who do not get pregnant, then after 6 months the pregnancy rate drops to < 10% month. On the other hand, when we look at data on unexplained infertility, the best predictor of outcome of treatment is duration of fertility. If we treat women with endometriosis, whatever the medical treatment, and we do not take the duration of infertility into account then it is impossible to draw any reliable results.

Dr Malinak

Dr Sibel from Boston studied danazol versus no treatment and found that the pregnancy rate was lower in the patients who received danazol when compared with those who received no treatment.

Prof. Schweppe

There are five or six other studies with comparative trials, danazol or medroxyprogesterone acetate, where there is no treatment. The problem is with the selection of patients and the design of the study. For example, if there is a group with endometriosis and a mean duration of, say, 3.4 years of infertility, it is very difficult to understand why, according to the data on the natural fertility rate just quoted by Prof. Koninckx, how a couple who have been unable to get pregnant after 3.5 years will get pregnant following diagnostic laparoscopy and biopsy for endometriosis and then just follow-up.

If it is necessary to do such a study we must start with no treatment for the whole group and then split them into two groups, treating one group with danazol and the other group randomized expectant management again. Then we shall get hard figures.

7

Combination medical–surgical therapy for endometriosis

L.R. Malinak and J.M. Wheeler

INTRODUCTION

Unfortunately, there is more speculation as to the value of perioperative medical therapy for endometriosis than there is data. The few studies on perioperative therapy are cohort studies, many of which are retrospective. Surgeons seem to 'believe' in either pre- or postoperative medical therapy, even though their own data does not suggest advantage of one method over the other. The even fewer prospective cohort studies on perioperative medical therapy are subject to selection bias due to the lack of randomized study group assignment. Also, many studies have an over-representation of milder cases, entering the possibility of spectral bias in any overall conclusions; certainly, analyses of combination therapy must be stratified by severity of disease by some measure (recognizing the imperfections in *all* current measures of severity!). Hopefully, recent randomized clinical trials comparing danazol and GnRH agonists will be followed for the 5 years necessary to gather meaningful recurrence data.

It is the frequency of recurrent endometriosis after medical or surgical therapy, and the documentation of microscopic endometriosis, that has brought the issue of combination therapy into the forefront of treatment options. Concomitant advances in medications (e.g. depot forms of GnRH agonists) and reproductive surgery (e.g. operative endoscopy) make a combination approach even more likely to be used in the immediate future.

The purpose of this paper is to review the current literature on combination therapy, as well as to outline the factors that make combination therapy theoretically sound. We conclude by calling for properly designed trials to answer finally the question as to whether pre- or post- or no perioperative treatment is preferable in treating endometriosis.

THEORETICAL REASONS FOR COMBINATION MEDICAL/SURGICAL THERAPY

Frequent recurrences with medical or surgical 'single agent' therapy

Many drugs have demonstrated efficacy in reducing the size of endometriosis implants, including danazol, progestins, androgens and GnRH agonists. Similarly, surgical treatment with coagulation, excision or vaporization reduces the number of endometriosis implants in the patient. However, the few long-term longitudinal cohort studies available document unacceptably high rates of recurrence with either medical or surgical treatment alone: typically, 5 year recurrence rates of 30–40% with either surgical or medical treatment are reported[1]. In addition to long-term recurrence, both medical and surgical treatments are associated with short-term recurrences – even though often clinically silent. Second-look laparoscopy studies have documented recurrent endometriosis just a few months after discontinuance of medical therapy or laparotomy. Despite these problems with short- and long-term recurrence, somatic symptoms improve and infertile couples regularly conceive after medical or surgical therapy alone. Clearly, our understanding of the natural history is biased by our surgical observations; we simply don't know 'how much' endometriosis treatment comprises adequate treatment. Furthermore, 'how much' treatment may depend upon the particular outcome in which we are interested. The recurrence data suggests that there is some threshold level of endometriosis above which pelvic pain or infertility results – it is not an 'all or none' phenomenon. The fact that mild endometriosis is found in 11% of asymptomatic women undergoing surgery unrelated to endometriosis suggests that the milder forms of this disease may be a variant of normal, rather than a pathological disease. This could certainly explain how *any* treatment – including expectant treatment – has a high pregnancy rate in infertile women with mild endometriosis. Thus, all endometriosis may not have to be eliminated to produce pregnancy, yet more complete treatment is more likely to reduce disease recurrence rates.

Presence of microscopic endometriosis

In addition to concern about recurrence, Murphy and colleagues documented microscopic endometriosis in about a quarter of grossly normal peritoneal biopsies in women with endometriosis elsewhere in the pelvis[2]. Some surgeons have questioned whether these microscopic implants are meaningful or not: certainly, we don't know enough about their natural history to conclude firmly whether microscopic disease progresses or regresses in most cases.

Varying vascular supply among endometriosis lesions

Along with high recurrence rates and known microscopic implants, a third fact that encourages the use of combination therapy is the varying vascularity between lesions. Medical treatment of ovarian endometriomata and fibrotic plaques is never successful: all medications seem dependent upon arriving at metabolically active implants via a rich blood supply due to the surrounding inflammation. The only exception to this may be intraperitoneal therapy – an area of interest to several groups including ours. Also, we are about to begin using transvaginal Doppler-aided sonography in evaluating differential blood flow to different areas in the pelvis in women with endometriosis when compared with controls. Clearly, avascular lesions must be removed surgically: preoperative medication may aid dissection, and postoperative medication may eliminate any residual macro- or microscopic disease.

Multifocal nature of endometriosis

Endometriosis is typically a multifocal disease. Whereas the occasional patient will have one large focus of endometriosis, most will have several or many areas of involvement. Surgical identification and removal/ destruction of all these lesions is difficult. Furthermore, endometriosis can occur following hysterectomy and oophorectomy – suggesting that whatever aetiological factors are operative may continue after traditional 'complete' therapy. Therefore, postoperative medical therapy may treat the entire mesothelium remaining, regardless of the extent of involvement.

LITERATURE OVERVIEW

Over ten years ago, Audebert and colleagues used 600–800 mg of danazol daily post-conservative laparotomy for 3–5 months in women with invasive ovarian disease[3]. A third of the patients conceived up to 34 months after therapy. These authors also prescribed preoperative danazol to 26 of the patients, of whom 42% conceived. This study was neither randomized nor standardized in terms of endometriosis classification.

The use of pseudopregnancy regimens was reported initially to be useful perioperatively[4], but later was found to be less efficacious than surgery alone[5]. More importantly, the side-effects of the pseudo-pregnancy regimen, coupled with the availability of other medications equally efficacious but with more tolerable side-effects, have caused pseudopregnancy to be virtually abandoned in most clinical centres.

We reported improved pregnancy rates in a small retrospectively collected cohort of women with severe endometriosis who were treated with post-laparotomy danazol for 3–6 months[6]. This study was then followed with prospective accrual of patients, although in a non-randomized fashion: improved pregnancy rates were seen in women with moderate and severe endometriosis[7].

Buttram and colleagues carried out a prospective comparision of preoperative and postoperative danazol[8]. Assignment was non-random, and more severe cases were entered into the postoperative danazol group. There was no statistical difference in recurrence rates between preoperative and postoperative therapy. Donnez has similarly reported his findings of better success with preoperative lynoestrenol[9].

Olive and Martin studied laser laparoscopic treatment of endometriosis alone and in combination with preoperative and postoperative danazol[10]. Using monthly fecundity as their outcome, they failed to demonstrate any consistent advantage of pre- or postoperative danazol. However, a small sample size seriously limits their statistical likelihood of demonstrating a difference – should one truly exist.

FUTURE RESEARCH

Clearly, this body of literature is so tenuous that well-planned randomized trials should be conducted to compare perioperative therapy with surgery alone. Such a trial would have to take into account the changing epidemiology of endometriosis towards a greater proportion of milder cases, as well as a greater likelihood of being treated via operative laparoscopy. Performance bias by the surgeons must be compensated for by a second observer, and assessment made of inter-rater reliability. The invalidity of current classifications can be overcome by detailed recording of the operative findings and by morphometric analysis[11]. The trial must have 'double dummy' placebos due to likely placebo effect on pain or possible pregnancy. It is apparent that the time has come for definitive study of this subject, due to the current confusion and large numbers of patients being treated empirically with expensive medication.

CONCLUSION

There is much more theoretical suggestion for combination medical/surgical treatment of endometriosis than there is data confirming its efficacy compared to single agent therapy. Whereas several excellent surgeon/investigators advocate preoperative therapy, there is no data to suggest preoperative is better than postoperative, and vice versa. However, most authors do advocate postoperative therapy in the worst of cases regardless of preoperative medication. The size of this problem, as well as the shortcomings of our knowledge, makes this an essential topic to be studied by randomized clinical trials.

REFERENCES

1. Wheeler, J.M. and Malinak, L.R. (1987). Recurrent endometriosis. In Bruhat, M. (ed). *Endometriosis: Proceedings of an International Symposium,*

pp. 13–21. (Basel: Karger)

2. Murphy, A.A., Green, W.R., Bobbie, D., dela Cruz, Z.C. and Rock, J.A. (1986). Unsuspected endometriosis documented by scanning electron microscopy in visually normal peritoneum. *Fertil. Steril.*, **46**, 522–4

3. Audebert, A.J.M., Larrue-Charlus, S. and Emperaire, J.C. (1979). Endometriosis and infertility: a review of 62 patients treated with danazol. *Postgrad. Med. J.*, **55**, 10–14

4. Andrews, W.C., (1980). Medical versus surgical treatment of endometriosis. *Clin. Obstet. Gynecol.*, **23**, 917–26

5. Hammond, C.B., Rock, J.A. and Parker, R.T. (1976). Conservative treatment of endometriosis: the effects of limited surgery and hormonal pseudopregnancy. *Fertil. Steril.*, **27**, 756–62

6. Wheeler, J.M., and Malinak, L.R. (1981). Postoperative danazol therapy in infertility patients with severe endometriosis. *Fertil. Steril.*, **36**, 460–3

7. Wheeler, J.M., Maccato, M.L. and Malinak, L.R. (1985). Postoperative danazol: pregnancy rates in women with endometriosis treated by combined conservative surgical therapy/immediate postoperative danazol. Presented at the *Annual Meeting of the American Fertility Society*, September, Chicago, Illinois

8. Donnez, J., Lemaire-Rubbers, M., Karaman, Y., *et al.* (1987). Combined (hormonal and microsurgical) therapy in infertile women with endometriosis. *Fertil. Steril.*, **48**, 239–42

9. Olive, D.L. and Martin, D.C. (1987). Treatment of endometriosis-associated infertility with CO_2 laser laparoscopy: the use of one- and two-parameter exponential models. *Fertil. Steril.*, **48**, 18–24

10. Olive, D.L. and Haney, A.F. (1986). Endometriosis-associated infertility: a critical review of therapeutic approaches. *Obstet. Gynecol. Surv.*, **41**, 538–50

11. Wheeler, J.M. and Malinak, L.R. (1987). Computer graphic pelvic mapping, second-look laparoscopy, and the distinction of recurrent vs. persistent endometriosis. Presented at the *Annual Meeting of the American Fertility Society*, September, Reno, Nevada

DISCUSSION

Prof. Koninckx

When I feel it is too difficult to excise endometriosis by laser I give preoperative treatment, and almost invariably I have difficulty at that time in finding the border between normal tissue and endometriotic tissue.

Dr Malinak

We have wondered about the same dichotomy of benefit. Clearly the vascularity around the disease is reduced because of preoperative medical therapy, whether it be danazol or the analogues. On the other hand, the appearance of the lesions is different and the adjacent tissues handling is different. What we do not know is if it benefits the patient.

Overall, most surgeons say that in severe disease ease of resection is improved, but I certainly appreciate the problem with preoperative medical therapy.

8

Endometriosis: the management of recurrent disease

J.L.H. Evers, G.A.J. Dunselman, J.A. Land and P.X.J.M. Bouckaert

INTRODUCTION

> *Macavity's a Mystery Cat: he's called the Hidden Paw —*
> *For he's the master criminal who can defy the Law.*
> *He's the bafflement of Scotland Yard, the Flying Squad's despair:*
> *For when they reach the scene of crime — Macavity's not there!*
>
> T.S. Eliot
> *Old Possum's Book of Practical Cats*

Everybody knows endometriosis, but no one knows what it is. The frequency of occurrence of active endometriosis in asymptomatic patients without fertility problems remains unknown. The natural course of the disease is a mystery. It has been suggested that only in one third of cases is the disease progressive, whereas in as much as 60% and more of cases the disease remains in a steady state, or eventually even resolves spontaneously. Only a few studies are available that describe the evolution of the disease in a prospective way, without medical or surgical intervention. Yet, if one is to deal with recurrence of the disease and its management, one should at least have insight into the nature of the disease process, and the factors that allow or restrain its development. Whereas retrograde menstruation apparently occurs on an almost monthly basis in the vast majority of ovulating women, only a fraction of them come to our attention, either because of pain, or because of infertility. Perhaps only a disturbance of the delicate balance between the monthly peritoneal insult of retrograde menstruation and the defence mechanisms in the abdominal cavity will allow the disease to take root and develop. Thereafter, the disease may exist (and persist, in spite of medical or surgical therapy) as invisible, microscopic foci which, depending on the circumstances, may progress into manifest disease. Although by surgical therapy one may remove all visible implants, and by medical therapy one may render all active implants inactive and hence invisible (due to the lack of sequelae: mucus, haemorrhage, inflammatory reaction), active microscopic foci may persist and progress again to active disease. Recurrence of disease therefore usually cannot be differentiated from expanding, previously microscopic, endometriotic implants.

A special – epidemiological – problem in judging the factual rate of recurrence is posed by the fact that the means which are applied to determine it are in most studies predominantly patient- and doctor-dependent. Few studies report, for example, performance of a second-look laparoscopy for documentation of follow-up results as part of a prospective study design. Others provide data based on recurrence of symptoms as a measure of recurrence of disease.

IS ENDOMETRIOSIS A PROGRESSIVE OR A SELF-LIMITING DISEASE?

More and more authors agree that an intra-abdominal steady state exists in which defence mechanisms (including leukocytes, macrophages, inflammatory response, encapsulation and sequestration, fibrosis) are operative that keep peritoneal insult (by regurgitated menstrual sludge) at bay, and prevent, in most patients, the implantation of viable menstrual cells in crevices of the peritoneal and ovarian surfaces. If the defence is defective or the offence too strong, regurgitated endometrial cells may implant and give rise to the development of a disease entity that is clinically recognised as endometriosis. The stage of development at which the disease can be controlled by the peritoneal defence mechanisms is as yet unknown, but it may very well be that even after clinically recognizable implants have appeared the defence may gain the upper hand and overpower the disease. On the other hand, if after medical suppression of the disease, or after surgical destruction of all the visible lesions, the defence mechanisms fail, the residual viable (microscopic) implants may regenerate, especially after resumption of ovarian activity. Also, reseeding due to resumed retrograde menstruation will contribute to reappearance of the disease after discontinuance of medical suppression of ovarian activity. Recurrent (or persistent) endometriosis will then be diagnosed.

The data from Thomas and Cooke is one of the very few studies reporting the natural evolution of the disease[1]. They performed laparoscopies in a group of 17 patients who did not receive treatment, before and after 6 months of taking placebo (Table 1). In eight patients progress of the disease process was observed, in three of whom the deterioration included the appearance of adhesions that resulted in ovarian enclosure. In nine patients the disease improved, or did not progress to such a degree that it became obvious in the 6 months interval between laparoscopies: it became completely invisible at second-look laparoscopy in four of these nine patients. No factor, including the original severity score of endometriosis, the age of the patient, her parity, the Quetelet index, or the duration of infertility, could accurately predict improvement or deterioration of the endometriosis in the placebo group.

Table 1 Numbers of patients showing elimination, improvement, or deterioration of endometriosis in a placebo treatment group[1]

	Patients	*Percentage*
Disease eliminated	4/17	24%
Disease improved	5/17	29%
Disease deteriorated	8/17	47%

Janssen and Russell were the first to report on the course of non-pigmented endometriosis[2]. In their group of 77 patients they had the opportunity to relaparoscope six patients who did not receive any form of treatment. Non-pigmented lesions had progressed to typical pigmented endometriotic stigmas in these six patients within the course of 6–24 months between laparoscopies. In their opinion this confirmed the existence of a continuum between non-pigmented and pigmented endometriotic lesions.

Further corroboration of the presumption of endometriosis being a progressive disease came from the work of Redwine[3] who, in a transverse study, found an age-related colour appearance of endometriotic lesions (Table 2). This would suggest a natural evolution from the fresh, clear, active and productive papules of early endometriosis to the old, black, fibrotic and inactive lesions that have always been described as powder-burn or tobacco-stained puckerings.

Table 2   Evolution of colour appearance of endometriosis with age: mean age of patients with respective lesions

Colour appearance	Mean age in years
Clear papules only	21.5
Clear lesions only	23.0
Clear plus any others	23.4
Red lesions only	26.3
Red plus any others	26.9
All non-black lesions	27.9
White plus any others	28.3
Black plus any others	28.4
White lesions only	29.5
Black lesions only	31.9

From Redwine[3]

When studying recurrence of endometriosis one should always keep in mind that medical therapy does most probably not eradicate endometriosis, and that by surgery one can only destroy the lesions which are visible to the eye (with or without a magnification provided by the laparoscope). We compared the number and the cumulative size of endometriotic implants before and after 6 months of treatment with danazol in two groups of patients[4]. In both groups the first-look laparoscopy was performed during the follicular phase of the cycle. In the first group the second-look laparoscopy (SLL) was performed at the end of the last treatment cycle; in the second group the SLL was performed in the follicular phase of the second spontaneous menstrual cycle after the end of treatment. A statistically significant reduction in the number and the cumulative size of the implants was found in the group with a SLL during ovarian suppression by danazol, but not in the group with a SLL after resumption of ovarian activity[4] (Figures 1 and 2). It was concluded that medical therapy does not eradicate endometriosis. If suppression is discontinued, the endometriotic lesions will regenerate with time.

REPORTS ON RECURRENCE OF ENDOMETRIOSIS AFTER THERAPY

Recurrence rates of endometriosis after conservative surgical treatment vary from 7–47%[5–9]. Wheeler and Malinak have determined long-term recurrence rates by means of a historical prospective study design coupled with life-table analysis (Figure 3)[10]. The fact that their curve representing the cumulative recurrence rate does not (yet) show the typical asymptotic deflection one would expect from survival curves, makes one speculate that endometriosis will eventually reappear in all patients who had their visible lesions removed at initial surgery. After all, it is not possible to remove all endometriotic lesions at the time of initial surgery. Even ablation of all the cul-de-sac peritoneum, as has been reported in this era of laser surgery, will lead to recurrence. Microscopic endometriotic microfoci will remain[11–13]. These may subsequently develop into visible endometriotic implants and present, together with new implants from reseeded endometrial cells, as recurrence of disease in these endometriosis-prone patients.

Recurrence figures of endometriosis after medical therapy vary from 29–51%[14–18]. The difference between the various recurrence rates reported may be explained by the difference in the length of follow-up, and by the difference in the way recurrence is diagnosed, i.e. by recurrence of symptoms of endometriosis, by laparoscopy with or without histological confirmation or by the need to perform a repeat laparotomy. Also, marker substances (e.g. anti-endometrial antibodies, CA-125) have been used to document recurrence[19]. Although the sensitivity of most of the markers described is too low to allow their use as a screening tool, they may have a place in the follow-up of patients with proven (and treated) endometriosis.

It is not clear whether the recurrence noted after cessation of therapy represents real recurrence, i.e. *de novo* formation, or rather persistence and

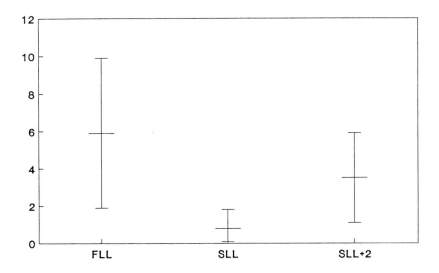

Figure 1 Number of endometriotic implants seen during first-look laparoscopy (FLL), as compared with the number of implants seen when second-look laparoscopy was performed during the last week of a 6 month treatment period with danazol (SLL) or during the follicular phase of the second spontaneous cycle after discontinuation of danazol treatment (SLL+2)[4]

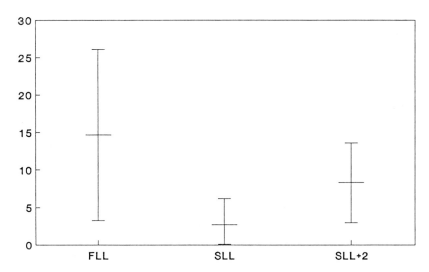

Figure 2 Cumulative diameter of endometriotic implants seen during FLL, as compared with the cumulative diameter seen during SLL and SLL+2 respectively[4]

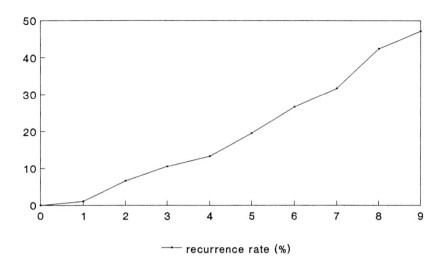

Figure 3 Long-term recurrence rate of endometriosis after conservative surgical therapy, as determined by means of a historical prospective study design coupled with life-table analysis [10]

reactivation of endometriotic lesions that had been rendered quiescent by medical suppression of ovarian hormonal activity. Biopsy specimens taken during repeat laparoscopy at the end of treatment repeatedly show occult inactive endometriosis [20] or active disease, even in the absence of laparoscopic (macroscopic) signs of endometriosis [12,21,22]. In a prospective study of 60 patients, Wheeler and Malinak [9] showed that in half of them so-called recurrence of endometriosis after conservative surgery actually represented persistence of disease and progression of previously invisible microfoci to visible implants. Schweppe showed that persistence of disease after 6 months of medical therapy was correlated with the histological differentiation of the endometriotic lesions at the initial diagnostic laparoscopy [23]. Of the highly differentiated endometriotic lesions, two thirds disappeared after 6 months treatment, whereas of the poorly differentiated lesions three-quarters persisted. It has to be kept in mind, as stated before, that since most of the second-look laparoscopies were performed during ovarian suppression and not during normal cyclic ovarian activity (as usually was the first-look laparoscopy during which the diagnosis was made), the results of medical therapy may be overestimated: implants are suppressed, regardless of the type of drug administered, but not eliminated[4,22,24,25]. This makes one wonder if most, if not all, of the recurrence should in fact better be defined as persistence of disease.

TREATMENT OF RECURRENT ENDOMETRIOSIS

From the above it can be concluded that no essential difference exists between primary and recurrent endometriosis, as far as therapeutic options are concerned. Recurrent endometriosis is either *de novo* formation in a patient who allowed development of the disease originally, or it is progression of previously invisible microfoci into visible implants after surgical or medical therapy. Therefore, the choice of treatment in a patient with recurrent endometriosis will not be determined by the manifestation of the disease as such (be it primary or recurrent), but by the extent of the pelvic disturbances, especially the distortion of the tubal–ovarian spatial relationships, and by the reason that made the patient seek medical help. In a patient who has a recurrence of endometriosis that interferes with her desire for fertility repeat conservative surgery has a favourable prognosis for conception. We found a 38% pregnancy rate among our eight patients undergoing repeat conservative surgery for endometriosis (Table 3). Seven of Wheeler and Malinak's 15 patients[10] (47%), and 29% of Ranney's patients[26] conceived after conservative re-operation. The average pregnancy rate of these series of re-operations is about 40%, which makes it a procedure to be taken into consideration when counselling a patient about her fertility prognosis.

Patients in whom the pelvic disturbances, due either to endometriosis or to postoperative adhesion formation following previous surgery, do not appear to allow successful reoperation should be offered assisted reproduction. *In vitro* fertilization (IVF) or one of its many derivatives, possibly after prior medical suppression of endometriotic activity, may offer such patients a fair chance of pregnancy[27].

Patients with symptomatic endometriosis but not desiring future fertility may be afforded relief by painkillers. If not, long-term hormonal therapy is indicated, in the form of cyclic birth-control pills or uninterrupted progestagen medication. The value of presacral

Table 3 Conservative surgery for endometriosis in infertility patients: results and recurrences in the Maastricht series

	n *Patients*	
Conservative surgery I[a]	42	
Pregnant	26	62%
Conservative surgery II	8	
Pregnant	3	38%
Conservative surgery III	1	
Pregnant	0	

a) I, II and III indicate first, second and third conservative operations performed on the same patient

neurectomy and of uterosacral nerve ablation in endometriosis–related pain has still to be determined.

If no wish for future fertility exists, and if medical and/or conservative surgical therapy have failed, definitive surgery may be indicated. It includes bilateral oophorectomy, resection of all endometriosis and/or hysterectomy. Hormone replacement therapy (HRT) should be started in the premenopausal patient, although in severe cases it is advisable to postpone treatment for an arbitrary period of at least 6 months. The risk of inciting regrowth of residual endometriosis after that time is negligible (see later). During the first 6 months following oophorectomy, oestrogen deprivation symptoms may be suppressed by progestins.

In conclusion, treatment of recurrent endometriosis should be tailored to the patient and her complaints, i.e. pain and/or infertility. Since probably most of the recurrent disease is evolution of microscopic disease, treatment does not necessarily have to differ from that in a patient with primary disease. In our clinics we employ a flowchart for those patients who have recurrent endometriosis, and whose stage of disease does not make them straightforward candidates for either assisted reproduction techniques or definitive surgery (Figure 4).

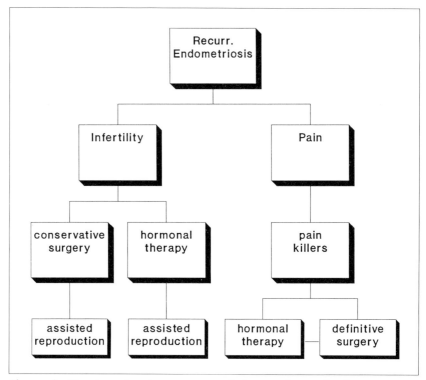

Figure 4 Flowchart for the treatment of those patients who have recurrent endometriosis, and whose stage of disease does not make them straightforward candidates for either assisted reproduction techniques or definitive surgery

REFERENCES

1. Thomas, E.J. and Cooke, I.D. (1987). Impact of gestrinone on the course of asymptomatic endometriosis. *Br. Med. J.*, **294**, 272–4
2. Janssen, R.P.S. and Russell, P. (1986). Nonpigmented endometriosis: clinical, laparoscopic, and pathologic definition. *Am. J. Obstet. Gynecol.*, **155**, 1160–3
3. Redwine, D.B. (1987). Age-related evolution on color appearance of endometriosis. *Fertil. Steril.*, **48**, 1060–3
4. Evers, J.L.H. (1987). The second-look laparoscopy for evaluation of the result of medical treatment of endometriosis should not be performed during ovarian suppression. *Fertil. Steril.*, **47**, 502–4
5. Green, T.H. (1966). Conservative surgical treatment of endometriosis.

Clin. Obstet. Gynecol., **9**, 293–308

6. Andrews, W.C. and Larsen, G.D. (1974). Endometriosis: treatment with hormonal pseudopregnancy and/or operation. *Am. J. Obstet. Gynecol.*, **118**, 643–51

7. Hammond, C.B, Rock, J.A. and Parker. R.T. (1976). Conservative treatment of endometriosis: the effects of limited surgery and hormonal pseudopregnancy. *Fertil. Steril.*, **27**, 756–66

8. Andrews, W.C. (1980). Medical versus surgical treatment of endometriosis. *Clin. Obstet. Gynecol.*, **23**, 917–24

9. Wheeler, J.M. and Malinak, L.R. (1987). Computer graphic pelvic mapping second-look laparoscopy and the distinction of recurrent versus persistent endometriosis. *Fertil. Steril. Progam suppl. 43rd Ann. Meeting.*, (abstract 194), p. 79

10. Wheeler, J.M. and Malinak, L.R. (1987). Recurrent endometriosis. *Contr. Gynecol. Obstet.*, **16**, 13–21

11. Acosta, A.A., Buttram, V.C. Jr., Besch, P.K., Malinak, L.R., Franklin, R.R. and Vanderheyden, J.D. (1973). A proposed classification of pelvic endometriosis. *Obstet. Gynecol.*, **42**, 19–25

12. Murphy, A.A., Green, W.R., Bobbie, D., Cruz, Z.C. de la and Rock, J.A. (1986). Unsuspected endometriosis documented by scanning electron microscopy in visually normal peritoneum. *Fertil. Steril.*, **46**, 522–4

13. Dmowski, W.P. (1987). Visual assessment of peritoneal implants for staging endometriosis: do number and cumulative size of lesions reflect the severity of a systemic disease? *Fertil. Steril.*, **47**, 382–4

14. Dmowski, W.P. and Cohen, M.R. (1978). Antigonadotropin (danazol) in the treatment of endometriosis. Evaluation of posttreatment fertility and three-year follow-up data. *Am. J. Obstet. Gynecol.*, **130**, 41–8

15. Greenblatt, R.B. and Tzigounis, V. (1979). Danazol treatment of endometriosis: longterm follow-up. *Fertil. Steril.*, **32**, 518–20

16. Dmowski, W.P. Kapetanakis, E. and Scommegna, A. (1982). Variable effects on endometriosis at 4 low dose levels. *Obstet. Gynecol.*, **59**, 408–15

17. Buttram, V.C. Jr. (1985). Treatment of endometriosis with danazol: report of a 6-year prospective study. *Fertil. Steril.*, **43**, 353–60

18. Schmidt, C.L. (1985). Endometriosis: a reappraisal of pathogenesis and treatment. *Fertil. Steril.*, **44**, 157–73

19. Kauppila, A., Telimaa, S., Ronnberg, L. and Vuori, J. (1988). Placebo-controlled study on serum concentrations of CA-125 before and after treatment of endometriosis with danazol or high-dose medroxyprogesterone acetate or after surgery. *Fertil. Steril.*, **49**, 37–41

20. Steingold, K.A., Cedars, M., Lu, J.K.H., Randle, D., Judd, H.J. and Meldrum, D.R. (1987). Treatment of endometriosis with a long-acting

gonadotrophin-releasing hormone agonist. *Obstet. Gynecol.*, **69**, 403–11

21. Dmowski, W.P. and Cohen, M.R. (1975). Treatment of endometriosis with an antigonadotropin, danazol: a laparoscopic and histologic evaluation. *Obstet. Gynecol.*, **46**, 147–54

22. Schweppe, K.W., Dmowski, W.P. and Wynn, R.N. (1981). Ultrastructural changes in endometriotic tissue during danazol treatment. *Fertil. Steril.*, **36**, 20–6

23. Schweppe, K.W. (1984). *Morphologie und Klinik der Endometriose*. pp. 198–207. (Stuttgart and New York: F.K. Schattauer Verlag)

24. Cornillie, F.J., Brosens, I.A., Vasquez, G. and Riphagen, I. (1986). Histologic and ultrastructural changes in human endometriotic implants treated with the antiprogesterone steroid ethylnorgestrinone (gestrinone) during two months. *Int. J. Gynecol. Path.*, **5**, 95-109

25. Cornillie, F.J., Puttemans, P. and Brosens, I.A. (1987). Histology and ultrastructure of human endometriotic tissues treated with dydrogesterone (Duphaston). *Eur. J. Obstet. Gynecol. Reprod. Biol.*, **26**, 39–55

26. Ranney, B. (1978). Re-operation after initial treatment of endometriosis with conservative surgery (discussion). *Am. J. Obstet. Gynecol.*, **131**, 416–21

27. Oehninger, S., Acosta, A.A., Kreiner,D., Mussler, S.J., Jones, H.W. Jr. and Rosenwaks, Z. (1988). *In vitro* fertilization and embryo transfer (IVF/ET): an established and successful therapy for endometriosis. *J. In vitro Fertil. Embryo Transf.*, **5**, 249–56

DISCUSSION

Prof. Donnez

Referring to your presentation, in cases of frequency of endometriosis in infertile women it was suggested that the patients be given hormonal therapy before assisted reproduction. I suppose that for assisted reproduction hMG and hCG would be administered. Could the administration of such drugs increase the severity of the disease?

Dr Evers

I do not know. There is a lot of evidence in endometriosis that by utilizing only super-ovulation we can obtain a reasonable pregnancy rate comparable to IVF figures in the patients with endometriosis.

Of course, no one has done laparoscopy before and after hMG and hCG which would be the way to answer your question.

Prof. Donnez

In cases of ovarian endometriosis, I think the pregnancy rate following IVF is lower than in the controls.

Dr Evers

Yes.

Dr Cornillie

The success of IVF when ovarian disease is present is less because many more cycles are cancelled. If during stimulation cyst formation is seen to occur, the cycle gets stopped. It does not necessarily have anything to do with less fertilization or less implantation, it is just that more cycles have to be cancelled.

I have a question for Dr Evers. It has been said many times that recurrence is not seen that frequently where pregnancies occur earlier. Is there any good data or is that just speculation? What can pregnancy do for endometriosis?

Dr Evers

The only way to study this is to have a very long-term follow-up. As far as I have found in the literature, what pregnancy does is to postpone recurrence. In the large studies with long-term follow-up there is recurrence, but it is later than in the group that did not achieve pregnancies.

Of course this is difficult reasoning. Those patients who achieve a pregnancy will be the patients whose disease is less severe, which makes the statistical analysis of the difference rather complicated.

9

Endometriosis and infertility: a continuing debate

E.J. Thomas

INTRODUCTION

Over the last 20 years there has been a large increase in the number of infertile patients found to have endometriosis. It is uncertain whether this represents an actual increase or is simply a reflection of the more frequent use of laparoscopy in the investigation of the infertile couple. This paper will investigate the relationship between pelvic endometriosis and infertility. The possible mechanisms by which the disease may cause infertility will be discussed and then the evidence that there is a causal relationship between the endometriosis and infertility will be reviewed. Finally, the vexed question of the role of medical treatment in endometriosis in infertility will be addressed.

THE RELATIONSHIP BETWEEN ENDOMETRIOSIS AND INFERTILITY

Most clinicians would agree that endometriosis which is associated with tubal or ovarian damage or with adhesion formation, will materially affect future fertility. Controversy, however, exists about the relationship between small amounts of asymptomatic endometriosis and infertility. It does appear that there is a relationship because endometriosis has been reported in up to 60% of women undergoing laparoscopy for infertility[1-3]. This compares with an incidence of 2.5–5% in fertile controls[1,4]. However, there is little evidence that this relationship is causal, and it is interesting to note that more recent publications have been reporting high incidences of endometriosis in women having sterilizations reversed[5,6]. This is a group in which it could be expected to find a very low incidence of the disease, especially as the tubes have been occluded. The explanation for the high incidence is probably the increased sensitivity of gynaecologists to making the visual diagnosis of endometriosis. Whilst this is the case, great care must be taken in interpreting reports of incidences in specific groups and especially in attributing causality to an apparant increase.

MECHANISMS THROUGH WHICH ENDOMETRIOSIS MAY CAUSE INFERTILITY

There have been six main mechanisms which have been postulated to cause infertility in women with endometriosis. These are:

(1)   reproductive endocrine abnormalities,

(2)   prostaglandin abnormalities,

(3)   dysfunction of peritoneal macrophages,

(4)   an altered immune response,

(5)   oocyte dysfunction,

(6)   increased abortion rate.

Reproductive endocrine abnormalities

Anovulation, disorders of gonadotrophin secretion, luteal phase defects, abnormalities of prolactin secretion and the luteinized unruptured follicle syndrome have all been investigated as causes of infertility in endometriosis. In the initial studies there appeared to be a high incidence of these abnormalities in infertile women with endometriosis[7-14]. In general, however, more detailed and controlled studies have provided conflicting information which shows no excess of these abnormalities[15–19]. Obviously this is a simplistic analysis of the published work, but detailed reading leads to the conclusion that there is no good evidence that there is an increased incidence of reproductive endocrine disorders in endometriosis above that to be expected in unexplained infertility.

Prostaglandin metabolism

As with endocrine abnormalities, the data about the importance of prostaglandins in infertility in endometriosis is conflicting. Investigations in both human and in animal models have shown differences in the concentration of prostaglandin E2 and F2-α in the peritoneal fluid in endometriosis[20–22]. There are, however, studies which have been unable to demonstrate these differences[23–25]. Whether the abnormalities are caused primarily by the endometriosis or are secondary to inflammation is not resolved. Furthermore, even if the abnormalities exist, there is no proof that they are causal in infertility. It is hypothesized that the high concentrations of these prostaglandins in peritoneal fluid may alter tubal motility or corpus luteum function, but there is no experimental evidence to show this *in vivo*.

Peritoneal macrophages

Peritoneal fluid contains leukocytes of which a majority are macrophages. Higher concentrations of these macrophages have been demonstrated consistently in patients with endometriosis when compared with normal controls or women with unexplained infertility[22,26,27]. These macrophages appear to be at higher activation[28,29] and phagocytose sperm more avidly than normal controls[30]. Recent reports have shown increased levels of interleukin-1 and macrophage-derived growth factor in the peritoneal fluid in endometriosis[31,32]. The relevance of this finding is unknown, but it is interesting to note that peritoneal fluid from endometriosis is more toxic to mouse embryos than that from controls[33]. There is, therefore, evidence to suggest that the peritoneal fluid in endometriosis is a hostile environment for gametes and embryos. However, there is no substantial evidence that this environment actually decreases fertility *in vivo*.

Abnormalities in immunity

Various early reports have shown diffuse abnormalities in immunoglobulins[34], cell mediated immunity[35] and autoantibodies[36] in women with endometriosis. More recent data have substantiated these[37-39]. It has been hypothesized that these abnormalities could affect implantation or the maintenance of the pregnancy. As with other postulated causes, there is little scientific evidence of these adverse effects *in vivo*. At present it is not possible to tell whether these immune phenomena are important in the pathogenesis of endometriosis and infertility or are secondary to the disease or its associated inflammation.

Oocyte dysfunction

An initial report by Wardle and colleagues showed that oocytes from women with endometriosis had a lower fertilization rate than those with tubal disease or unexplained infertility on an *in vitro* fertilization (IVF) programme[40]. However, since then the majority of reports have not shown lower fertilization or pregnancy rates on IVF and gamete intrafallopian transfer (GIFT) programmes in women with endometriosis[41,42], which would suggest that oocyte dysfunction is unlikely to play a major role in infertility in endometriosis.

Abortions

A number of retrospective studies have shown a higher incidence of first trimester abortions in women with endometriosis than would be expected in the normal population[43-45]. There is a dearth of prospective, controlled studies and a recent report concluded that the high abortion rates can be explained by factors other than endometriosis[46]. Further evidence in support of this is provided by Regan and colleagues who demonstrate in a prospective study that it is a women's previous reproductive performance that is the most important factor in determining whether a pregnancy miscarries[47]. It is, therefore, unlikely that abortions constitute a major cause of infertility in endometriosis, but proper studies need to be mounted.

Overall, there is conflicting evidence that any of the mechanisms described above are causal in the infertility associated with endometriosis. In order to investigate this causality further, the appropriate analysis is to observe whether the treatment of the disease results in improved fertililty.

RESULTS OF TREATMENT OF ENDOMETRIOSIS IN INFERTILITY

There are many uncontrolled studies in the literature which have shown high pregnancy rates after the treatment of endometriosis, both surgically and medically. However, the scientific weakness of uncontrolled studies is well established and this section will only review prospective controlled studies. The first study to use a non–treatment control group in comparison with danazol in infertile women with endometriosis showed a lower cumulative conception rate (CCR) in the treatment group (36%) than in the controls (47%)[48]. This difference was not statistically significant. The numbers in the study were increased and reported in 1988[49]. This showed CCR at 12 months of 37% in the danazol group and 57% in the controls. This difference was not statistically different ($p < 0.1$) but certainly could not demonstrate a benefit of treatment. This absence of benefit has been further shown in studies comparing danazol with expectant management[50] and with medroxyprogesterone acetate[51].

There are only two studies which have compared treatment to placebo. Telimaa compared 18 patients on danazol with 17 on medroxy-progesterone acetate and 14 on placebo[52]. The CCRs at 30 months were 33%, 42% and 46% respectively. Thomas and Cooke compared 20 patients treated with gestrinone for 6 months against 17 treated with placebo, and they reported CCR at 12 months of 25% and 30% respectively[53]. In conclusion, these studies could not demonstrate a benefit to future fertility by treating endometriosis which has not caused tubo-ovarian adhesions or tubal blockage. Because of the small numbers of patients in the studies, it cannot be assumed that endometriosis does not have a partial impact on future fertility.

THE ROLE OF TREATMENT OF ENDOMETRIOSIS IN INFERTILIITY

The reviews in this paper have been unable to demonstrate good evidence that endometriosis causes infertility *in vivo*. They have also been unable to show a causal role for the disease in controlled treatment studies. It must, therefore, be asked if there is a role for treatment of endometriosis in infertility especially as current therapies are potently contraceptive and can have unpleasant side-effects. Obviously symptomatic disease should be treated, but there is no obvious reason to treat asymptomatic disease unless it can be demonstrated that harm occurs by not so treating. A knowledge of the natural history of the disease would help in this assessment and there are two studies which have performed placebo-controlled trials in which the placebo group received a second laparoscopy after 6 months. Telimaa and colleagues showed resolution of the disease in only 18% of those on placebo and deterioration in 23%[54]. Thomas and Cooke showed improvement in five out of 17 patients on placebo with deterioration in eight (47%)[55]. In both studies there was significantly less improvement and significantly more deterioration if the disease was untreated. Therefore, it appears that there is a need to treat asymptomatic endometriosis in order to avoid deterioration and the appearance of peri-tubal or peri-ovarian adhesions which was reported by Thomas and Cooke[55]. However, recent evidence of the temporary effect of drug therapy[56] questions the certainty of the necessity to treat. Obviously if the disease returns to its pretreatment state in a percentage of women it is not logical to continue treating them permanently in order to avoid deterioration. Perhaps electro-coagulation at the time of laparoscopy for small amounts of endometriosis is the preferred treatment. It means that there is no delay in attempting conception and no drug side-effects. Recent evidence showing a superior pregnancy rate in endometriosis treated by laparoscopic diathermy against expectant management supports this[57]. In the end these dilemmas will only be resolved when there is more investigation into the pathogenesis and natural history of the disease.

REFERENCES

1. Hasson, H.M. (1976). Incidence of endometriosis in diagnostic laparoscopy. *J. Reprod. Med.*, **16**, 135–8
2. Goldenberg, R.L. and Magendantz, H.G. (1976). Laparoscopy and the infertility evaluation. *Obstet. Gynecol.*, **47**, 410–14
3. Drake, T.S. and Grunert, G.M. (1980). The unsuspected pelvic factor in the infertility investigation. *Fertil. Steril.*, **34**, 27–31
4. Strathy, J.H., Molgaard, C.A., Coulam, C.B. and Melton, L.J. (1982). Endometriosis and infertility: a laparoscopic study of endometriosis among fertile and infertile women. *Fertil. Steril.*, **38**, 667–72
5. Fakih, H.N., Tamura, R., Kesselman, A. and De Cherney, A. (1985). Endometriosis after tubal ligation. *J. Reprod. Med.*, **30**, 939–41
6. Dodge, S.T., Pumphrey, R.S. and Miyazawa, K. (1986). Peritoneal endometriosis in women requesting reversal of sterilization. *Fertil. Steril.*, **45**, 774–7
7. Soules, M.R., Malinak, L.R., Bury, R. and Poindexter, A. (1976). Endometriosis and anovulation: a co-existing problem in the infertile female. *Am. J. Obstet. Gynecol.*, **125**, 412–15
8. Dmowski, W.P., Cohen, M.R. and Wilhelm, J.L. (1976). Endometriosis and ovulatory failure: Does it occur? Should ovulatory stimulating agents be used? In Greenblatt, R.B. (ed). *Recent Advances in Endometriosis.* pp. 129–36. (Amsterdam: Excerpta Medica, International Congress Series)
9. Cheeseman, K.L., Ben-nun, I., Chatterton, R.T. and Cohen, M.R. (1982). Relationship of luteinizing hormone, pregnendiol -3- glucuronide and estriol -16- glucuronide in urine of infertile women with endometriosis. *Fertil. Steril.*, **38**, 542–8
10. Grant, A. (1966). Additional sterility factors in endometriosis. *Fertil. Steril.*, **17**, 514–19
11. Hargrove, J.T. and Abraham, G.E. (1980). Abnormal luteal function in endometriosis. *Fertil. Steril.*, **34**, 302
12. Hirschowitz, J.S., Soler, N.G. and Wortsman, J. (1978). The galactorrhoea–endometriosis syndrome. *Lancet*, **1**, 896–8
13. Brosens, I.A., Koninckx, P.R. and Corvelyn, P.A. (1978). A study of plasma progesterone, oestradiol-17β, prolactin and LH levels, and of the luteal phase appearance of the ovaries in patients with endometriosis and infertility. *Br. J. Obstet. Gynecol.*, **58**, 246–50
14. Lesorgen, P.R., Wu, C.H., Green, P.J., Gocial, B. and Lerner, L.J. (1984). Peritoneal fluid and serum steroids in infertility patients. *Fertil. Steril.*, **42**, 237–42
15. Radwanska, E. and Dmowski, W.P. (1981). Luteal function in infertile

women with endometriosis. *Infertility*, **4**, 269–77

16. Pittaway, D.E., Maxson, W., Daniell, J., Herbert., C. and Wentz, A.C. (1983). Luteal phase defects in infertility patients with endometriosis. *Fertil. Steril.*, **39**, 712–13

17. Muse, K., Wilson, E.A. and Jawad, M.J. (1982). Prolactin hyperstimulation in response to thyrotropin-releasing hormone in patients with endometriosis. *Fertil. Steril.*, **38**, 419–22

18. Dmowski, W.P., Rao, R. and Scommegna, A. (1980). The luteinized unruptured follicle syndrome and endometriosis. *Fertil. Steril.*, **33**, 30–34

19. Dhont, M., Serryn, R., Duvivier, P., Vanluchene, E., De Boevor, J. and Vanderkerkhove, D. (1984). Ovulation stigma and concentration of progesterone and oestradiol in peritoneal fluid: relation with fertility and endometriosis. *Fertil. Steril.*, **41**, 872–7

20. Schenken, R.S., Asch, R.J., Williams, R.F., and Hodgen, G.D. (1984). Etiology of infertility in monkeys with endometriosis. Luteinized unruptured follicles, luteal phase defects, pelvic adhesions and spontaneous abortions. *Fertil. Steril.*, **41**, 122–30

21. Drake, T.S., O'Brien, W.F., Ramwell, P.W. and Metz, S.A. (1981). Peritoneal fluid thromboxane B2 and 6-keto prostaglandin F1 alpha in endometriosis. *Am. J. Obstet. Gynecol.*, **140**, 401–4

22. Badawy, S.Z.A., Cuenca, V., Marshall, L., Munchback, R., Rinas, A.C. and Coble, D.A. (1984). Cellular components in peritoneal fluid in infertile patients with and without endometriosis. *Fertil. Steril.*, **42**, 704–8

23. Rock, J.A., Dubin, N.H., Ghodgaonkar, R.B., Bergquist, C.A., Erozan, Y.S. and Kimball, A.W. (1982). Cul-de-sac fluid in women with endometriosis: fluid volume and prostanoid concentrations during the proliferative phase of the cycle – days 8 to 12. *Fertil. Steril.*, **35**, 747–50

24. Sgarlata, C.S., Hertelendy, F. and Mikhail, G. (1983). The prostanoid content in peritoneal fluid and plasma of women with endometriosis. *Am. J. Ostet. Gynecol.*, **147**, 563–5

25. Rezai, N., Ghodgaonkar, R.B., Zacur, H.A., Rock, J.A. and Dubin, N.H. (1987). Cul-de-sac fluid volume, protein and prostanoid concentration during the peri-ovulatory period – days 13 to 17. *Fertil. Steril.*, **48**, 29–32

26. Haney, A.F., Muscato, J.J. and Weinberg, J.B. (1981). Peritoneal fluid cell populations in infertility patients. *Fertil. Steril.*, **35**, 696–8

27. Halme, J., Becker, S., Hammond, M.G. and Ray, S. (1982). Pelvic macrophages in normal and infertile women: the role of patent tubes. *Am. J. Obstet. Gynecol.*, **142**, 890–5

28. Halme, J., Becker, S., Hammond, M.G., Ray, M.H.G., and Ray, S. (1983). Increased activation of pelvic macrophages in women with mild endometriosis. *Am. J. Obstet. Gynecol.*, **145**, 333–7

29. Halme, J., Becker, S. and Haskill, S. (1987). Altered maturation and function of peritoneal macrophages: possible role in pathogenesis of endometriosis. *Am. J. Obstet. Gynecol.*, **156**, 783–9

30. Muscato, J.J., Haney, A.F. and Weinberg, J.B. (1982). Sperm phagocytosis by human peritoneal macrophages: a possible cause of infertility in endometriosis. *Am. J. Obstet. Gynecol.*, **144**, 503–10

31. Halme, J., White, C., Kauma, S., Estes, J. and Haskill, S. (1988). Peritoneal macrophages from patients with endometriosis release growth factor activity *in vitro. J. Clin. Endrocinol. Metab.*, **66**, 1044–49

32. Fakih, H., Baggett, B., Holtz, G., Tsang, K.Y., Lee, J.C. and Williamson, H.O. (1987). Interleukin-1: a possible role in the infertility associated with endometriosis. *Fertil. Steril.*, **47**, 213–7

33. Morcos, R.N., Gibbons, W.E. and Findley, W.E. (1985). Effect of peritoneal fluid on *in vitro* cleavage of 2-cell mouse embryos: possible role in infertility associated with endometriosis. *Fertil. Steril.*, **44**, 678–83

34. Weed, J.C. and Arquembourg, P.C. (1980). Endometriosis: can it produce an autoimmune response resulting in infertility? *Clin. Obstet. Gynecol.*, **23**, 885–91

35. Steele, R.W., Dmowski, W.P. and Marmer, D.J. (1984). Immunologic aspects of human endometriosis. *Am. J. Reprod. Immunol.*, **6**, 33–6

36. Mathur, S., Peress, M.R., Williamson, H.O. *et al.* (1982). Autoimmunity to endometrium and ovary in endometriosis. *Clin. Exp. Immunol.*, **50**, 259–66

37. Meek, S.C., Hodge, D.D. and Musich, J.R. (1988). Autoimmunity in infertile patients with endometriosis. *Am. J. Obstet. Gynecol.*, **158**, 1365–73

38. Hill, J.A., Faris, H.M., Schiff, I. and Anderson, D.J. (1988). Characterization of leukocyte subpopulations in the peritoneal fluid of women with endometriosis. *Fertil. Steril.*, **50**, 216–22

39. Badawy, S.Z., Cuenca, V., Stitzel, A. and Tice, D. (1987). Immune rossettes of T and B lymphocytes in infertile women with endometriosis. *J. Reprod. Med.*, **32**, 194–7

40. Wardle, P.G., McLaughlin, E.A., McDermott, A. *et al.* (1985). Endometriosis and ovulatory disorder: reduced fertilization *in vitro* compared with tubal and unexplained infertility. *Lancet* **ii**, 236–9

41. Wong, P.C., Ng, S.C., Hamilton, M.P. *et al.* (1988). Eighty consecutive cases of gamete intra-fallopian transfer. *Hum. Reprod.*, **3**, 231–3

42. Yovich, J.L., Matson, P.L., Richardson, P.A. and Hilliard, C. (1988). Hormonal profiles and embryo quality in women with severe endometriosis treated by *in vitro* fertilization and embryo transfer. *Fertil. Steril.*, **50**, 308–13

43. Petersohn, L. (1970). Fertility in patients with ovarian endometriosis before

and after treatment. *Acta. Obstet. Gynec. Scand.*, **49**, 331–3

44. Naples, J.D., Batt, R.E. and Sadigh, H. (1981). Spontaneous abortion rate in patients with endometriosis. *Obstet. Gynecol.*, **57**, 509–12

45. Olive, D.L., Franklin, R.R. and Gratkins, D. (1982). The association between endometriosis and spontaneous abortion. *J. Reprod. Med.*, **27**, 333–8

46. Pittaway, D.E., Vernon, C. and Fayez, J.A. (1988). Spontaneous abortion in women with endometriosis. *Fertil. Steril.*, **50**, 711–15

47. Regan, R., Braude, P.R. and Trembath, P.L. (1989). Influence of past reproductive performance on risk of spontaneous abortion. *Br. Med. J.*, **299**, 541–5

48. Seibel, M.M., Berger, M.J., Weinstein, F.G. and Taymor, M.L. (1982). The effectiveness of danazol on subsequent fertility in minimal endometriosis. *Fertil. Steril.*, **38**, 534–7

49. Bayer, S.R., Seibel, M.M., Saffan, D.S., Berger, M.J. and Taymor, M.L. (1988). Efficacy of danazol treatment for minimal endometriosis in infertile women. *J. Reprod. Med.*, **33**, 179–83

50. Badawy, S.Z., El Bakry, M.M., Samuel, F. and Dizer, M. (1988). Cumulative pregnancy rates in infertile women with endometriosis. *J. Reprod. Med.*, **33**, 757–60

51. Hull, M.E., Moghissi, K.S., Magyar, D.F. and Hayes, M.F. (1987). Comparison of different treatment modalities in infertile women with endometriosis. *Fertil. Steril.*, **47**, 40–4

52. Telimaa, S. (1988). Danazol and medroxyprogesterone acetate inefficacious in the treatment of infertility in endometriosis. *Fertil. Steril.*, **50**, 872–5

53. Thomas, E.J. and Cooke, I.D. (1987). Successful treatment of endometriosis: does it benefit infertile women? *Br. Med. J.*, **294**, 1117–9

54. Telimaa, S., Puolakka, J., Ronnberg, L. and Kauppila, A. (1987). Placebo-controlled comparison of danazol and high-dose medroxyprogesterone acetate in the treatment of endometriosis. *Gynecol. Endocrinol.*, **1**, 13–23

55. Thomas, E.J. and Cooke, I.D. (1987). Impact of gestrinone on the course of asymptomatic endometriosis. *Br. Med. J.*, **294**, 272–4

56. Evers, J. (1987). The second-look laparoscopy for the evaluation of the results of medical treatment should not be performed during ovarian suppression. *Fertil. Steril.*, **47**, 502–4

57. Nowroozi, K., Chase, J.S., Check, J.H. and Wu, C.H. (1987). The importance of laparoscopic coagulation of mild endometriosis in infertile women. *Int. J. Fertil.*, **32**, 442–4

DISCUSSION

Dr Cornillie

We have a major problem in evaluating the effect of therapy using the American Fertility Society classification. It really does not reflect what is happening at a cellular level in the ectopic implants. It is more or less a visual inspection of the sequelae of the disease.

Dr Thomas

While I take Dr Cornillie's criticisms, and they are very valid, about using the American Fertility Society's system, in the end if we are to look at some sort of progress of the disease in a sensible clinical situation we have to use some scoring system, though none to date are perfect, particularly when infertility is being evaluated.

10

Medical management of mild endometriosis associated with infertility

G.B. Candiani, L. Fedele, P. Vercellini, S. Bianchi and L. Arcaini

INTRODUCTION

The true incidence of infertility in women with endometriosis is not known[1]. Although a direct cause-and-effect relationship between minimal and mild endometriosis and infertility has not been definitely established, numerous authors consider that pharmacological and/or surgical treatment may improve the reproductive prognosis[2]. A laparotomy to eliminate cirumscribed lesions seems excessive, and in the absence of periadnexal adhesions medical treatment would be more appropriate[3]. Clinical observations and experimental data suggest that steroid hormones are the major growth and function regulators of endometriotic tissue[4]. In the 70s and 80s numerous attempts have been made to treat mild endometriosis by pharmacological suppression of ovarian activity[4]. During the same period, however, reports have been published on women treated expectantly in whom the pregnancy rates were not inferior to those in patients receiving pharmacological or surgical treatment[5]. We analyzed the results of three pharmacological treatments, danazol, gestrinone and buserelin, administered to infertile women with mild endometriosis, and made comparison with a control group of women who did not take any drug. Thus we hoped to ascertain the most effective clinical approach in achieving a pregnancy.

MATERIALS AND METHODS

The series consisted of 115 women with infertility who in the period of 1985–88 underwent laparoscopy as a result of which minimal or mild endometriosis was diagnosed according to the revised American Fertility Society classification[6]. Prelaparoscopic investigations included a hysterosalpingography, evaluation of basal body temperature, evaluation of blood levels of progesterone and prolactin during the midluteal phase, a premenstrual endometrial biopsy, seminal analysis of the partner and a post-coital test. Women with bilateral tubal occlusion, pelvic adhesions, or severe systemic or endocrine disease were excluded from the study as were women who had received steroid treatment in the previous 6 months or whose partners had abnormal semen parameters. Women with multifactorial infertility were included only if the factors coexisting with endometriosis (e.g. ovulation defect, mild male factor) were limited and correctable. All the laparoscopies were performed by two of the authors under general endotracheal anaesthesia with a 10 mm diameter $0°$ diagnostic laparoscope (Olympus Optical Co. model A 5214) and an ancillary probe inserted in the suprapubic area. Although in some patients a biopsy was performed for histological confirmation of endometriosis, unipolar cautery or lasers were not used to eliminate the lesions. After the diagnosis the patients were allocated to one of the following treatments: danazol 200 mg three times a day for 6 months ($n = 41$), gestrinone 2.5 mg twice weekly for 6 months ($n = 13$), intranasal buserelin 400 mg three times daily for 6 months ($n = 32$), or expectant management ($n = 29$). Danazol was increased to 800 mg daily and gestrinone to 2.5 mg three times weekly if breakthrough bleeding occurred. This was not a controlled randomized trial since assignment of the patients to the different treatment groups was based on each woman's wish to receive medical therapy and on the type of drug being used in the clinic at the time of diagnosis. The women given expectant management were enrolled throughout the study period. The medical treatments were started the first day of the cycle after laparoscopy. After 6 months of treatment the patients were followed for a period varying from 8 to 40 months (mean = 16).

Data on recovery of fertility were analyzed with the life-table method. The groups were compared by χ-square analysis.

RESULTS

At the diagnostic laparoscopy, endometriosis was classified as Stage I in 62 patients and Stage II in 53. The mean age, parity, duration of infertility, and extent of the disease did not differ significantly among the four treatment groups (Table 1). Despite the high frequency of side-effects (Table 2), all the patients who received medical treatment completed the prescribed treatment period. In the blood tests performed at the end of 6 months of treatment, two patients in the danazol group presented a rise in serum aspartate aminotransferase and alanine aminotransferase which resolved spontaneously. Another woman in the same group reported deepening of her voice.

Although the women treated expectantly showed the best results in terms of reproductive recovery, the cumulative pregnancy rates at 18 months did not demonstrate significant differences among the four treatment groups (Table 3) nor when the patients with Stage I disease were compared with those in Stage II. The infertility co-factors additional to endometriosis, which were uniformly distributed in the four groups, were all corrected and thus did not influence the pregnancy rates. Also, in the evaluation of the monthly fecundity rates (MFR) no significant differences were found among the various treatment groups (Table 3). Life-table analysis of the four groups is shown in Figure 1.

Table 1 Clinical data of 115 patients with minimal or mild endometriosis

Treatment groups	No. of patients	Age (mean ± SD)	No. of parous patients	Months of infertility (mean ± SD)	R-AFS Stage* I	II
Danazol	41	30.8 ± 4.1	3	47.9 ± 23.4	21	20
Gestrinone	13	28.6 ± 3.9	–	52.3 ± 14.7	6	7
Buserelin	32	30.1 ± 3.7	2	40.4 ± 27.6	17	15
Expectant management	29	31.3 ± 4.8	4	54.1 ± 35.7	18	11

*The American Fertility Society. (1985). Revised American Fertility Society classification of endometriosis[6]

Table 2 Side-effects reported during medical treatments

	Danazol		Gestrinone		Buserelin	
	no.	*%*	*no.*	*%*	*no.*	*%*
Weight gain	29	70.7	6	46.2	3	9.4
Hot flushes	10	24.4	–	–	30	93.8
Vaginal dryness	4	9.8	–	–	12	37.5
Decreased breast size	9	21.9	1	7.7	7	21.9
Headache	5	12.2	2	15.4	9	28.1
Acne	10	24.4	3	23.1	–	–
Seborrhoea	9	21.9	2	15.4	–	–
Hirsutism	4	9.8	–	–	–	–
Muscle cramps	9	21.9	3	23.1	–	–
Nausea	6	14.6	1	7.7	1	3.1
Decreased libido	4	9.8	1	7.7	5	15.6
Deepening of voice	1	2.4	–	–	–	–
Increase of liver transaminases	2	4.9	–	–	–	–
Depression	4	9.8	1	7.7	3	9.4

Table 3 Recovery of fertility in 115 women with minimal or mild endometriosis

Treatment groups	No. of patients	Pregnancies				
		No.	Crude rate	Corrected rate	Cumulative rate[a]	MFR★
Danazol	41	16	39%[b]	47%[c]	44%[d]	0.029[e]
Gestrinone	13	4	31%[b]	40%[c]	34%[d]	0.030[e]
Buserelin	32	14	44%[b]	54%[c]	48%[d]	0.033[e]
Expectant management	29	15	52%[b]	60%[c]	54%[d]	0.041[e]

a: Cumulative pregnancy rates at 18 months follow-up
b, c, e: Not significant by χ-square analysis
d: Not significant by life-table analysis
★: Monthly Fecundity Rate

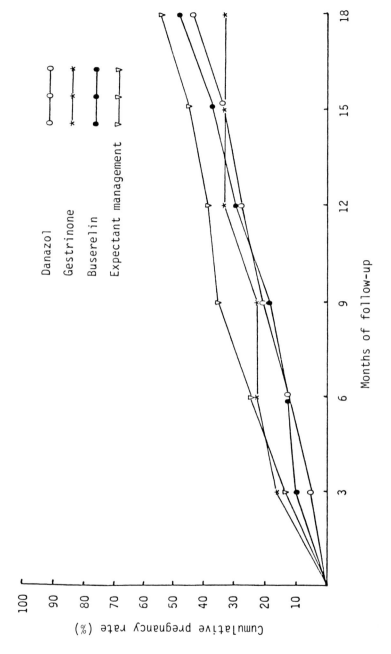

Figure 1 Cumulative pregnancy rates for the four treatment groups over an 18-month follow-up period

DISCUSSION

The efficacy of treatments for infertile women with mild endometriosis can be demonstrated only by prospective randomized studies including control groups and with adequate follow-up and correct statistical evaluation of the results[5]. Most clinical trials reported in the literature do not fulfil these prerequisites. In women with mild endometriosis treated consecutively the incidence of spontaneous pregnancy is far from negligible (Table 4). The pregnancy rates reported after conservative surgery,[7–9] danazol,[9–14] gestrinone[15] and GnRH agonists[16] do not seem significantly different from those obtained after simple observation[7,8,10,11,14,17–19].

The usefulness of our results is limited by the non–random allocation to the treatment groups and by the small number of women in each group. Each woman was carefully investigated to exclude other absolute or uncorrectable infertility factors in addition to endometriosis. Chi-square analysis demonstrated a homogeneous distribution of other confounding variables in the different groups. Staging was performed by only two observers. We did not perform a follow-up laparoscopy at 6 months of treatment. In fact, a repeat laparoscopic assessment at the end

Table 4 Expectant management for patients with infertility and mild endometriosis reported in the literature

Reference	No. treated	No. pregnant	Overall %	MFR*
Garcia and David, 1977[7]	17	11	64.7	0.050
Schenken and Malinak, 1982[8]	18	13	72.2	0.102
Siebel *et al.*, 1982[10]	28	14	50.0	0.111
Portuondo *et al.*, 1983[17]	31	19	61.2	0.083
Olive *et al.*, 1985[18]	34	13	52.9	0.057
Hull *et al.*, 1987[14]	56	21	37.5	
Bayer *et al.*, 1988[11]	36	17	47.2	
Present study, 1989	29	15	51.7	0.041
Total	249	129	53.0	

*Monthly Fecundity Rate

of pharmacological treatment is not necessarily a good index of successful resolution of the disease[20]. Furthermore, persistence of endometriotic lesions does not appear to affect the reproductive results[15].

Our control group consisted of the women who, during the study period, refused medical treatment. Although the best crude, corrected and cumulative pregnancy and monthly fecundity rates were observed in these patients, χ-square testing and life-table analysis did not demonstrate any statistically significant difference among the four treatment groups.

In two prospective randomized studies the cumulative pregnancy rate at 12 months was evaluated. This was 37.2% in 37 women with minimal endometriosis treated with danazol compared with 57.4% in 36 controls (p = NS) in Bayer and colleagues' study,[11] and 25% in 20 patients treated with gestrinone and 24% in 17 controls in the second study[15]. Henzl and colleagues, using 400 or 800 ug/day intranasally of nafarelin, a GnRH agonist, obtained similar pregnancy rates to those patients treated with danazol (30%, 52% and 36% respectively)[16].

After simple observation in infertile women with mild endometriosis, Portuondo and colleagues reported a cumulative pregnancy rate of 61.2% at 18 months[17], Olive and colleagues an overall pregnancy rate of 52.9%[18], and Rodriguez–Escudero and colleagues a cumulative pregnancy rate of 47.5% at 12 months[19]. These data suggest there is no real relation between minimal and mild endometriosis and infertility or that therapies based on an erroneous concept have been used which do not affect the pathogenetic mechanism(s) of endometriosis-associated infertility. Thomas and Cooke failed to show that the elimination of endometriosis after medical treatment had an impact on future fertility; according to these authors a diagnosis of mild endometriosis in infertile women is irrelevant since the cumulative pregnancy rates are the same in patients with unexplained infertility[15].

During medical treatment endometriotic lesions manifest glandular involution and stromal atrophy, but they persist in quiescent form with prompt regrowth at the resumption of ovarian activity[21,22]. Moreover, scanning electron microscope studies have demonstrated active endometriosis in visually normal peritoneal biopsies[23]. It has not been proven that the presence of ovarian hormones is the only or the main aetiological mechanism, and there may be a biological predisposition to the development of endometriosis. If this is the case, modifying the steroid environment for some months would be inappropriate therapeutic strategy. The correction of ovulation abnormalities, which are frequently associated with mild endometriosis, could resolve persistent infertility in many cases[24].

The results of the present study confirm that danazol, gestrinone and intranasal buserelin are ineffective in improving spontaneous reproductive prognosis of infertile women with minimal and mild endometriosis. The treatments used by us presented frequent and severe side-effects, and at least in Italy their cost is very high.

In 1977 Francis M. Ingersoll wrote: "A hazard of laparoscopy is that it may demonstrate either minimal pelvic inflammatory disease or a tiny spot of endometriosis for which no therapy is required. However, after the surgeon informs the apprehensive patient that she has endometriosis, she will ask questions or consult a textbook and find that endometriosis is associated with infertility, which will be a constant source of worry for her. She will seek other opinions, take any sort of prophylactic hormonal therapy, and even insist upon extirpating surgery, which is a much greater threat to her fertility than the minimal disease seen."[25] It seems to us that the mass of data reported in the literature in the intervening 12 years does not modify Ingersoll's view based on clinical experience.

REFERENCES

1. Burns, W.N. and Schenken, R.S. (1989). Pathophysiology. In Schenken, R.S. (ed.). *Endometriosis, Contemporary Concepts in Clinical Management*. pp. 83–126. (Philadelphia: J.B. Lippincott)
2. Muse, K. (1987). Endometriosis and infertility. In Wilson, E.A. (ed.)., *Endometriosis*. pp. 91–110. (New York: Alan R. Liss)
3. Wilson, E.A. (1988). Surgical therapy for endometriosis. *Clin. Obstet. Gynecol.*, **31**, 857–65
4. Barbieri, R.L. and Hornstein, M.D. (1987). Medical therapy for endometriosis. In Wilson, E.A. (ed.), *Endometriosis*. pp. 111–140. (New York: Alan R. Liss)
5. Olive, D.L. and Haney, A.F. (1986). Endometriosis-associated infertility: a critical review of therapeutic approaches. *Obstet. Gynecol. Survey*, **41**, 538–55
6. The American Fertility Society. (1985). Revised American Fertility Society Classification of Endometriosis. *Fertil. Steril.*, **43**, 351–2
7. Garcia, C.R. and David, S.S. (1977). Pelvic endometriosis: infertility and

pelvic pain. *Am. J. Obstet. Gynecol.*, **129**, 740–7

8. Schenken, R.S. and Malinak, L.R. (1982). Conservative surgery versus expectant management for the infertile patient with mild endometriosis. *Fertil. Steril.*, **37**, 183–6

9. Guzick, D.S. and Rock, J.A. (1983). A comparison of danazol and conservative surgery for the treatment of infertility due to mild or moderate endometriosis. *Fertil. Steril.*, **40**, 580–4

10. Seibel, M.M., Berger, M.J., Weinstein, F.G. and Taymor, M.L. (1982). The effectiveness of danazol on subsequent fertility in minimal endometriosis. *Fertil. Steril.*, **38**, 534–7

11. Bayer, S.R., Seibel, M.M., Saffan, D.S., Berger, M.J. and Taymor, M.L. (1988). Efficacy of danazol treatment for minimal endometriosis in infertile women. A prospective randomized study. *J. Reprod. Med.*, **33**, 179–83

12. Badawy, S.Z.A., El Bakry, M.M., Samuel, F. and Dizer, M. (1988). Cumulative pregnancy rates in infertile women with endometriosis. *J. Reprod. Med.*, **33**, 757–60

13. Butler, L., Wilson, E., Belisle, S., Gibson, M., Albrecht, B., Schiff, I and Stillman, R. (1984). Collaborative study of pregnancy rates following danazol therapy of stage I endometriosis. *Fertil. Steril.*, **41**, 373–6

14. Hull, M.E., Moghissi, K.S., Magyar, D.F. and Hayes, M.F. (1987). Comparison of different treatment modalities of endometriosis in infertile women. *Fertil. Steril.*, **47**, 40–4

15. Thomas, E.J. and Cooke, I.D. (1987). Successful treatment of asymptomatic endometriosis: does it benefit infertile women? *Br. Med. J.*, **294**, 1117–9

16. Henzl, M.R., Corson, S.L., Moghissi, K., Buttram, V.C., Beravist, C. and Jacobson, J. (1988). Administration of nasal nafarelin as compared with oral danazol for endometriosis. A multicenter double-blind comparative clinical trial. *N. Engl. J. Med.*, **318**, 485–9

17. Portuondo, J.A., Echanojauregni, A.D., Herran, C., and Alijarte, I. (1983). Early conception in patients with untreated mild endometriosis. *Fertil. Steril.*, **39**, 22–5

18. Olive, D.L., Stohs, G.F., Metzger, D.A. and Franklin, R.R. (1985). Expectant management and hydrotubations in the treatment of endometriosis-associated infertility. *Fertil. Steril.*, **44**, 35–41

19. Rodriguez Escudero, F.J., Neyro, J.L., Corcostegni, B. and Benito, J.A. (1988). Does minimal endometriosis reduce fecundity? *Fertil. Steril.*, **50**, 522–4

20. Evers, J.L.H. (1987). The second-look laparoscopy for evaluation of the result of medical treatment of endometriosis should not be performed during ovarian suppression. *Fertil. Steril.*, **47**, 502–4

21. Nisolle-Pochet, M., Casanas-Roux, F. and Donnez, J. (1988). Histologic study of ovarian endometriosis after hormonal therapy. *Fertil. Steril.*, **49**, 423–6

22. Fayez, J.A., Collazo, L.M. and Vernon, C. (1988). Comparison of different modalities of treatment for minimal and mild endometriosis. *Am. J. Obstet. Gynecol.*, **159**, 927–32

23. Murphy, A.A., Green, W.R., Bobbie, D., dela Cruz, Z.C. and Rock, J.A. (1986). Unsuspected endometriosis documented by scanning electron microscopy in visually normal peritoneum. *Fertil. Steril.*, **46**, 522–4

24. Doody, M.C., Gibbons, W.E. and Buttram, V.C. (1988). Linear regression analysis of ultrasound follicular growth series: evidence for an abnormality of follicular growth in endometriosis patients. *Fertil. Steril.*, **49**, 47–51

25. Ingersoll, F.M. (1977). Selection of medical or surgical treatment of endometriosis. *Clin. Obstet. Gynecol.*, **20**, 849–64

DISCUSSION

Prof. Donnez

I believe that peritoneal and ovarian endometriosis are not identical diseases, and when we are discussing infertility and endometriosis there are two different groups of patients: patients with mild and patients with minimal endometriosis. I would agree that the disease is then enigmatic as far as explaining infertility is concerned and that for the patient with moderate and severe endometriosis it means ovarian endometriosis, and that in this group probably the endometriosis causes infertility.

Prof. Vercellini

If we look at the studies published in the literature, I could find no single proof that any kind of treatment, whether medical treatment of any kind or laser treatment, has any benefit in terms of fertility. I am also not sure that the presence of minimal or mild endometriosis has been adequately evaluated in the fertile population. There are several reports in the literature that show that minimal and mild endometriosis when looked for properly are probably much more prevalent than is assumed.

We cannot exclude the hypothesis that minimal endometriosis is an ubiquitous disease and that sometimes, in advanced form, it can affect fertility.

Prof. Donnez
It is important to specify that Professor Vercellini is speaking only of minimal and mild endometriosis.

Dr Thomas
There has been recent evidence in rabbits with ovarian endometriosis that we see much less ovulation that we do in experimental endometriosis on the peritoneum. So possibly it might be site dependent.

Dr Cornillie
The question is no longer whether mild or minimal disease cause infertility. The question is what is the natural history of these minimal lesions, and should we treat them?

As Dr Thomas has shown, if there is a natural history of progression to moderate or severe disease, then there is a place for treatment, even surgical treatment. But the task is now in the hands of the morphologists and the pathophysiologists to tell the clinicians what the natural history really is and what is the real origin and the evolution of the disease. And that will need a considerable amount of basic work.

Prof. Shaw
In this last session we have been trying to evaluate the relationship between mild/moderate disease and infertility, and certainly we have questioned very much the value of any treatment in this situation except to prevent progression in the future.

11

A retrospective study of oestrogen replacement therapy following hysterectomy for the treatment of endometriosis

A.F. Henderson, J.W.W. Studd and N. Watson

INTRODUCTION

Endometriosis is the commonest gynaecological surgical abnormality encountered today following uterine leiomyomata. It is established that 2–3% of the white female population in their reproductive years are affected, and that endometriosis causes 40% of all infertility except that related to male factors[1]. Recurrence rates of 16–52% following treatment are reported at 1 year depending on the method of diagnosis and type of treatment[2]. There is also a residual 10–20% of patients in whom the disease fails to improve with any of the standard hormonal treatments available[3]. Medical treatments may be associated with metabolic and symptomatic side-effects and have limited effect in controlling symptoms due to adhesive disease or damaged pelvic organs. Conservative surgery with minimal disruption of the reproductive organs is obviously relevant where fertility is still of primary concern. However, a retrospective study has shown that this approach is associated with a cumulative recurrence rate of endometriosis in 13% of patients at 3 years and 40% at 5 years[4].

Preservation of ovarian tissue even at hysterectomy is still frequently employed in the belief that it produces reasonable cure rates[5-7]. Our previous study suggests that this approach is far from satisfactory in preventing recurrent symptoms with over 45% of patients requiring further surgery[8]. The preservation of ovarian tissue at surgery even in older women[9] may be due to several reasons. There may be a reluctance to inflict an acute premature menopause on patients with the possible concomitant long-term sequelae[10], but this need only apply if the patient is denied the proven benefits of hormone replacement therapy[11]. There may also be fears of a recurrence of the disease following oestrogen therapy, given that endometriosis is a condition driven by cyclical ovarian activity. However, previous studies have already indicated that oestrogen therapy is not contraindicated in women following hysterectomy for endometriosis[8,12-15]. The rationale behind this approach is further discounted by recent evidence of the steadily progressive nature of the disease in all patients[16]. This contradicts the generally held belief that there is no significant association between patient age and severity of the disease[17].

In view of these conflicting facts we have conducted a retrospective study to evaluate the role of hysterectomy, oophorectomy and hormone replacement therapy in the management of endometriosis.

PATIENTS AND METHODS

A retrospective study of 109 women with endometriosis treated by hysterectomy and hormone replacement implants was carried out. 115 women were contacted by postal questionnaire (47 replied; 40% response) and by telephone interview (62 contacted; 55% response). Six women were lost to follow-up. Information was obtained regarding age, parity, duration of the disease, method of diagnosis, duration and nature of medical and surgical treatment, and the state of the pelvis at the final laparotomy. The women were also questioned about their attitudes to hysterectomy and oophorectomy, and the effect of hormone therapy on their endometriosis and climacteric symptoms.

Implants of 50 or 75 mg oestradiol with 100 mg testosterone were given as an out-patient procedure under local anaesthetic in the manner described by Thom and Studd[18]. The mean duration of treatment was 5.3 years (range 0.3–18 years). Mean oestradiol levels were 810 pmol/l (range 105–2100 pmol/l) and mean testosterone levels were 1.4 nmol/l (range

0.4–3.1 nmol/l). At the time of the questionnaire 106 of the 109 women remained on hormone replacement therapy. The mean age at the time of the study was 46.9 years and the mean duration of endometriosis was 11.4 years (Table 1). Of the cases, 47 (40%) were diagnosed by laparoscopy and 62 (60%) at laparotomy. In 68 patients the diagnosis was made at the time of hysterectomy.

Table 1   Endometriosis study

	Mean	Range
Age at time of study	46.9	32–68
Age at onset of endometriosis symptoms	32.8	13–63
Age at diagnosis of endometriosis	35.5	15–67
Age at first laparotomy	37.5	16–64
Age at hysterectomy	39.5	23–67
Age at bilateral oophorectomy (88 patients)	39.7	23–64

Medical treatment had been prescribed in 100 women for a mean duration of 6.8 years. This included danazol (17.4%), progestagens (27.5%), oral contraceptives (33.0%), GnRH analogues (0.9%), simple analgesics and heat treatment (12.8%) or none (8.4%).

Surgical procedures had been carried out at other hospitals in 53 women, hence precise operative and pathological details were not available in these cases. Histories in the 109 women indicated that 70 (64.2%) had one laparotomy prior to commencing hormone therapy, while the remaining 39 (35.8%) had multiple operations (Table 2). The mean age at hysterectomy was 39.5 years (range 23–67 years) and at bilateral oophorectomy was 39.7 years (range 23–64 years).

The patients formed two main groups depending on whether or not ovarian tissue was present at commencement of implant therapy. Eighty-five women (78%) had no residual ovarian tissue and the remaining 24 women (22%) had some residual tissue. Of the 85 women with no residual ovarian tissue, 53 (63.3%) had had a total hysterectomy and bilateral oophorectomy as the primary surgical procedure for endometriosis. The remaining 32 women (37.6%) required two or more operations to complete the removal of ovarian tissue prior to commencing hormone therapy (Table 2). Of the 24 women with ovarian tissue present, seven (29%) underwent two or more operations prior to commencement.

Table 2 Number of laparotomies prior to commencement of HRT

No. laparotomies	No ovarian tissue at commencement HRT		Residual ovarian tissue at commencement HRT	
1	53★		17	
2	18		4	
3	6	37.6%	2	29.2%
> 3	8		1	
Total	85	(78%)	24	(22%)

★ TAH + BSO as primary surgical procedure

RESULTS

The follow-up of these two groups revealed significant differences in outcome. The group of 85 women with no residual ovarian tissue was followed up for a mean of 5.3 years (range 0.5–18 years). Only one patient required a further operation after commencing implant therapy; this was a ureteric re-implantation which followed nine previous laparotomies (Table 3). All the other women had excellent improvement in endometriosis symptoms, particulary pelvic pain and dyspareunia, and had no appreciable climacteric symptoms.

The group of 24 women with residual ovarian tissue at commencement of implant therapy was followed for a mean of 3.4 years (range 0.25–8 years). Six women (25%) required further laparotomies during this period for apparent recurrence of endometriosis symptoms, mainly pelvic pain (Table 4). Four women required one further laparotomy each: two had bilateral oophorectomy and two had division of adhesions. Two women required two further laparotomies each: one had sub-acute bowel obstruction secondary to adhesions, and one had a bilateral oophorectomy in two stages. No visible or histological evidence of recurrence of the endometriosis was found in any patient at repeat laparotomy.

Table 3 No ovarian tissue at commencement of oestrogen therapy

	No. patients	Mean age	Mean duration oestrogen (years)	Laparotomies following oestrogen
One operation (TAH + BSO)	53	49.8 (31–68)	5.5 (0.5–16)	0
More than one operation	32	45.7 (32–68)	5.2 (0.5–18)	1★

★ Ureteric re-implantation following nine laparotomies

Table 4 Ovarian tissue at commencement of oestrogen therapy

	No. patients	Mean age	Mean duration oestrogen (years)	Laparotomies following oestrogen
One operation (TAH alone)	17	46.6 (36–55)	3.7 (0.5–8)	4
More than one operation	7	46.5 (42–54)	3.1 (0.25–6.5)	2

There was no advantage to be gained by delaying implant therapy after oophorectomy in the group with no residual ovarian tissue. Of the 85 women in this group, 75 had immediate hormone replacement without any adverse effects. The remaining 10 women had a mean delay of 3.5 years (range 0.5–10 years) with predictable menopausal symptoms in the interim period. These symptoms were successfully treated with implants.

The attitudes of the women to hysterectomy and oophorectomy were notably different. Only five women (4.6%) had expressed any regrets about hysterectomy at the time of the operation but none had continuing regrets at the time of the study. Only one woman (aged 32, and nulliparous) had long-term retrospective regrets still present at the time of the study. However, 75 women (62.4%) had expressed reluctance to undergo bilateral oophorectomy at the time of hysterectomy. This was not significantly affected by parity or the number of previous operations, but was significantly related to the age at hysterectomy ($p < 0.01$) (Table 5).

Table 5   Attitude to oophorectomy at time of hysterectomy

	No.	Mean age at hysterectomy	Mean parity	No. operations
Happy/ no preference	34	41.7	1.2	2.8
Unhappy	75	37.3	1.2	2.3
Overall	109	39.5	1.2	2.5
Significance		< 0.01	ns	ns

ns = no significance

CONCLUSIONS

As expected in a condition which commonly affects the ovaries and is linked to cyclical ovarian activity, the results of this study suggest that repeated surgery is frequently necessary for control of symptoms until the last ovarian remnant is removed. This confirms the findings of our earlier study[9]. Thus in both groups of women, regardless of the state of ovarian tissue present at commencement of hormone therapy, a history of multiple operations was common. Of the 109 women overall, prior to commencing hormone therapy, two or more laparotomies had been performed in 39 cases (35.8%) and nine women (8.3%) had undergone four or more laparotomies. In the group of 85 women with no residual tissue, 32 women (37.6%) had undergone two or more operations for control of symptoms prior to commencing implants. Similarly, in the group of 24 women with residual tissue, seven (29.2%) had undergone two or more operations.

Significant differences in the outcome of the two groups appeared during the follow-up period of the study. In the former group, without ovarian tissue, none of the women required further surgery related to the return of endometriosis symptoms. In the latter group, however, a further six women (25%) underwent one or more subsequent operations to resolve persistent symptoms. No evidence of recurrence of endometriosis was found at repeat laparotomy in any of these patients, and the recurrence of symptoms was presumed to be due to adhesions or to 'residual ovary syndrome'. Furthermore, oestrogen replacement therapy did not increase the incidence of repeat laparotomy in this group: the incidence of multiple operations was 25% during the study compared to 29.2% prior to commencement of implants. Thus oestrogen replacement does not stimulate progression of the disease, and the risk of recurrent surgical intervention is likely to remain until complete surgery (i.e. total hysterectomy, bilateral oophorectomy and removal of endometriotic deposits) has been carried out.

No benefits are to be gained from delaying hormone replacement treatment following definitive surgery. Indeed, implants placed in the wound at closure provide a convenient role of administration and prevent the distressing and unnecessary climacteric symptoms suffered by the 10 women in this study.

Thus in cases of endometriosis where fertility is no longer of primary concern, the wisdom of early hysterectomy, bilateral oophorectomy, and immediate hormone replacement therapy is evident. Despite the reluctance shown by the majority of the women in this study to undergo bilateral oophorectomy, the patient can be reassured that this approach is effective in relieving both the symptoms and the progression of the disease, thus avoiding the pitfalls of repeated medical therapies and conservative surgery.

REFERENCES

1. Schweppe, K.-W. (1988). Etiology, pathogenesis and natural history of endometriosis. In Genazzani, A.R., Petraglia, F., Volpe, A. and Facchinetti, F. (eds.). *Advances in Gynecological Endocrinology*, Volume 2, pp. 79–96. (Carnforth: Parthenon Publishing)
2. Schmidt, C.L. (1985). Endometriosis: a reappraisal of pathogenesis and treatment. *Fertil. Steril.*, **44**, 157–73
3. Thomas, E.J. (1988). New perspectives in hormonal therapy for endometriosis. In Genazzani, A.R., Petraglia, F., Volpe, A. and Facchinetti, F. (eds.). *Advances in Gynecological Endocrinology*, Volume 2,

pp. 139–48. (Carnforth: Parthenon Publishing)

4. Wheeler, J.H. and Malinak, L.R. (1983). Recurrent endometriosis: incidence, management and prognosis. *Am. J. Obstet. Gynecol.*, **146**, 247

5. Ranney, B. (1971b). Endometriosis III. Complete operations. *Am. J. Obstet. Gynecol.*, **109**, 1137–44

6. Wilson, E.A. (1988). Surgical therapy for endometriosis. *Clin. Obstet. Gynecol.*, **31 (4)**, 857–65

7. Ranney, B. (1970). Endometriosis I: Conservative operations. *Am. J. Obstet. Gynecol.*, **107**, 743–53

8. Montgomery, J.C. and Studd, J.W.W. (1987). Oestradiol and testosterone implants after hysterectomy for endometriosis. In Bruhat, M.A and Canis, M. (eds.). *Contributions to Gynaecology and Obstetrics*, Volume 16, pp. 241–6. (Basel: Karger)

9. Elstein, M. and Bancroft, K. (1988). Endometriosis: the goal of treatment. In Genazzani, A.R., Petraglia, F., Volpe, A. and Facchinetti, F. (eds.). *Advances in Gynecological Endocrinology*, Volume 2, pp. 107–114. (Carnforth: Parthenon Publishing)

10. Studd, J.W.W. and Thom, M.H. (1981). Ovarian failure and ageing. *Clin. Endocrinol. Metab.*, **10**, 89–113

11. Whitehead, M.I. and Studd, J.W.W. (1988). Selection of patients for treatment: which therapy and for how long? In Studd, J.W.W. and Whitehead, M.I. (eds.). *The Menopause*. pp. 116–29. (London: Blackwell)

12. Studd, J.W.W., Andersen, H.M. and Montgomery, J.C. (1986). Selection of patients – kind and duration of treatment. In Greenblatt, R.C. (ed.). *A Modern Approach to the Perimenopausal Years*, pp. 129–40. (Berlin: Walter de Gruyter)

13. Hammond, C.B., Rock, J.A. and Parker, R.T. (1976). Conservative treatment of endometriosis; the effects of limited surgery and hormonal pseudopregnancy. *Fertil. Steril.*, **27**, 756–66

14. Dmowksi, W.P. (1981). Current concepts in the management of endometriosis. *Obstet. Gynecol. Ann.*, **10**, 279–311

15. Andrews, W.C. and Larson, G.D. (1974). Endometriosis: treatment with hormonal pseudopregnancy and/or operation. *Am. J. Obstet. Gynecol.*, **118**, 643–51

16. Thomas, E.J. and Cooke, I.D. (1987). Successful treatment of symptomatic endometriosis: does it benefit fertility? *Br. Med. J.*, **294**, 117–9

17. Buttram, V.C. and Betts J.W. (1979). Endometriosis. *Curr. Prob. Obstet. Gynecol.*, **2**, 3–58

18. Thom, M.H. and Studd, J.W.W. (1980). Hormonal implantation. *Br. Med. J.*, **280**, 848–50

DISCUSSION

Prof. Shaw

Obviously we do not have the information on whether there was active disease at the time of definitive surgery. Secondly, would the results have been any different if the patients had not been given testosterone? Is it in fact the testosterone that is preventing recurrence?

Dr Henderson

The reason we gave testosterone in most of the women was because of their young age. We find in our menopause clinic that testosterone is required for control of libido, it gives energy and it helps prevent depression. So from the point of view of carrying out a prospective controlled study there may be various ethical reasons for not giving it.

The testosterone levels in all the women were well within the normal range, and if there had been any suppressant effect of the testosterone implants we would have expected to see a lower incidence of repeat surgery in the group who still had residual ovarian tissue. But in that group there was no evidence that the hormone replacement therapy reduced the incidence of repeat surgery or the recurrence of symptoms. So I do not think the testosterone plays a major role.

Prof. Donnez

I have something of a similar opinion to Professor Shaw. I think that testosterone probably plays a role. I have the impression that in my patients treated by oestrogens alone following hysterectomy and oophorectomy for endometriosis they come back with more severe disease 2 or 3 years later. Also, I should like to ask whether you observed any androgenic side-effects.

Dr Henderson

Very few have androgenic effects, probably less than 0.5% stop testosterone implants because of androgenic side-effects. The vast majority obtain a considerable amount of beneficial side-effects.

Dr Malinak

Two aspects of treatment that are current in our community. First, at the time of hysterectomy and oophorectomy for severe endometriosis, if active disease is present at the time we withhold oestrogen replacement therapy for a period of time, arbitrarily 3–6 months, and during that time we would use Depo-provera or oral Provera as a method of preventing hot flushes and osteoporosis.

Second comment. Women in our community are very reluctant to give up their ovaries. Therefore if the ovaries are not involved, and particularly in younger women, the practice has been to preserve some ovarian function as long as the blood supply to that ovary is good and there is no ovarian involvement.

Dr Henderson
There is no evidence that any benefits are gained from delaying oestrogen therapy. Indeed, the 10 women in our study who were denied immediate treatment suffered severe menopausal symptoms. Progestagens will not control flushes adequately and are not a satisfactory treatment.

12

Issues of study design and statistical analysis in endometriosis research

J.M. Wheeler

INTRODUCTION

Endometriosis affects millions of women world-wide, and effectively employs tens of thousands of clinicians in its treatment and research. Certainly, clinicians, patients and related biomedical companies are all keenly interested in research that will advance our ability to manage endometriosis better. However, resources for research are limited – all questions surrounding endometriosis cannot be answered by randomized clinical trials (RCTs). Furthermore, all RCTs are not created equal: randomization and prospective data collection do not guarantee clinically meaningful results – witness the nafarelin study by Henzl and colleagues[1] that demonstrated for the first time ever that medical treatment for endometriosis can cause concomitant pelvic adhesions actually to disappear!

The tenets of clinical epidemiology – the science of clinical research study design – are just beginning to impact on endometriosis research. Previous studies have relied upon statisticians with limited clinical understanding of endometriosis to make critical decisions regarding study design. Clearly, both statisticians and clinicians will benefit from the 'translation' of one group's research concerns to the other group's vocabulary, and vice versa. To achieve this goal, this clinical essay reviews some of the study design and statistical issues that should be resolved prior to expenditure of millions of dollars on studies that will raise more questions than answers. Four of these key issues in endometriosis research are now outlined.

Patient accrual and cohort assembly

The standard list of inclusion and exclusion criteria fails to recognize our limited understanding of the natural history of endometriosis. Are women presenting with somatic symptoms the same as those presenting with infertility? Is their disease similar either in its mechanism of causing symptoms, its extent, or its likelihood of progression (or regression)? Other potential confounding factors that could seriously affect a fair comparison between cohorts include patient age, heritable versus spontaneous cases, and concomitant endocrinopathy such as anovulation or androgen excess. Statistically, these factors should not be assumed to simply 'wash out' with randomization schedules. Stratification is impractical; matching is possible on a few factors only. Multivariate methods could quantify these confounders, as well as unknown factors, at study conclusion.

Disease classification

Empirically-derived classification systems have, for 30 years, failed to produce a validated method of accurately predicting response to treatment. The most useful part of the currently widely used revised AFS system is its recommendation for a detailed drawing of operative findings: one solution to the lack of validated classification systems is the use of a detailed topographic record of pelvic pathology pre- and post-treatment, which we have termed 'pelvic mapping'. Only by the prospective collection of operative data in women with sufficient follow-up will meaningful classifications evolve.

Additional concerns with classification systems extend into statistical analysis. The rAFS system appears to be a linear scale, i.e. amenable to comparison of point scores by parametric tests. Yet, have we demonstrated that the five points difference between 50 and 45 is of the same importance as the same increment between 15 and 10 points? If we compensate for this invalid use of tests (assuming continuous data) by referring only to categorical Stages, have we demonstrated that Stage II is actually different enough from Stage I to merit its distinction as a separate category?

Finally, the current theory behind classification systems may be totally wrong. Do all types of implants – regardless of colour, associated inflammation, or invasiveness – count the same based just on size? Does implant size or location have anything to do with the mechanisms causing symptoms, particularly infertility? Is endometriosis a 'linear' disease as assumed by current classifications? Our data, along with others, suggest that there are not three or four separate categories of endometriosis, but rather an overlapping of a bimodal disease: a 'good endometriosis' group that responds to just about any therapy, including none at all, and a 'bad endometriosis' group, characterized by adhesions, invasiveness and frequent recurrence.

Susceptibility bias – endometriosis populations may vary in their susceptibility to cure by medical or surgical means

Medical therapy requires delivery of drug to the implant by the bloodstream: if differences in regional blood flow exist between individual patients, or within patients, erroneous conclusions could be reached comparing 'failures' with 'successes' that simply reflect variations in blood flow.

Surgical therapy requires removal of sufficient disease to affect the mechanism by which symptoms were produced. The likelihood of complete surgical treatment is likely affected by the depth of invasion, extent of unrecognized spread, association with microscopic implants, and location in relation to vital structures like the ureters. If these differences are sufficiently large between cohorts, erroneous conclusions could be reached regarding which patients have 'recurrent' implants after treatment.

Performance bias

Surgeons like to do surgery. Placebo controls, double-blinding, and assurances to equalize follow-up between cohorts is imperative for a fair comparison between the treatments performed.

To summarize thus far, numerous sources of bias are possible in clinical studies of endometriosis that may seriously distort the reliability of conclusions. Expensive RCTs should be based on sufficient pilot studies to answer some of these concerns, and use techniques that will minimize bias as much as possible. Although the 'perfect study' has not and will never be invented, it is our reponsibility to optimize our ability to interpret future studies to our patients and colleagues.

STATISTICAL METHODS IN ENDOMETRIOSIS RESEARCH

The most common calculations used in the clinical literature are crude or 'adjusted' pregnancy rates – most typically, annual pregnancy rates. This method is simple, and makes sense to patient and physician alike. However, these rates do not control for confounding factors either at baseline state (e.g. anovulation, male factor) or during the performance of the study manoeuvre. This method is going to be seen less often in research, to be relegated to conversation and discussion of clinical studies instead.

Monthly fecundity has the advantage of including a smaller unit of reported time (month) versus annual rates, and thus adds a certain degree of precision. Also, for comparison purposes, we know the monthly fecundity of normally fertile human couples is 0.21 per month. One major disadvantage, however, is the underlying statistical assumption that one time period (i.e. each month) is independent from all other time periods: clearly, especially with endometriosis treatment or recurrence, there is linkage from one month to the next.

Life-table analysis is much in vogue in presenting data from studies of infertility. The major advantage of life-table analysis is that each patient contributes to the overall results exactly that period of time for which she is clinically followed. In addition to being visually appealing in presenting data, there are both parametric and non-parametric methods for comparing two or three life-table curves. However, there is one underlying statistical assumption that does not seem to fit the application of life-tables to endometriosis: that there is a constant hazard function, meaning that from 1 month to the next, there is the same likelihood of conceiving. Clinically, we know that the vast majority of women who successfully conceive will do so within the first year after surgery.

Methods under development include categorical methods such as factor analysis that do not assume study parameters (e.g. disease classification) to be linear, continuous data. Multiple regression analysis is a robust enough statistical method to allow analysis of linear and ordinal variables, and allows one to control for multiple confounding factors. On the other hand, multiple regression is difficult for patients and physicians to understand, and requires large numbers of patients to perform.

CONCLUSION

Concomitant with improvements in the technologies of medical and surgical treatment of endometriosis is improvement in methodology of clinical research into this enigmatic disease. Future trials must, however, include as many effective measures as possible to reduce the potential for bias. Also, the various statistical methods available must be compared within existing groups of patients to compare their ability to give a realistic representation of trial results, yet control for distortion due to confounding factors, baseline differences, or variation in recording operative data.

REFERENCES

1.   Henzl, M.R., Corson, S.L., Moghissi, K., Buttram, V.C., Bergquist, C. and Jacobson, J. (1988). Administration of nasal nafarelin as compared with oral danazol for endometriosis. A multicenter double-blind comparative clinical trial. *N. Engl. J. Med.*, **318**, 485–9

DISCUSSION

Dr Dowsett

Could Dr Wheeler explain the statistical benefit for mismatching of numbers when he is guessing for a winner in the first instance? He was saying that if he feels that the LHRH agonist is likely to be better then he puts in perhaps two or three times as many. Does this shorten the trial?

Does it reduce the number of patients?

Dr Wheeler
Yes, and yes. There are different strategies in clinical trialling to try to shorten the trial, and one of them is betting on what is likely to win. So putting more patients in that group over the course of time makes that difference more apparent and the trial can be shortened. This has been seen in many different trials in many different fields over the last 30 years.

Prof. Donnez
Nothing was said about the multicentre study. What does Dr Wheeler think about that? There is another possibility of error.

Dr Wheeler
There are whole books written on the problems and advantages of muliticentre studies. The biggest advantage of multicentre studies is that populations vary. We Americans are a hodge-podge of peoples from all over the world and we may be different with our endometriosis. We are certainly different in terms of other things such as our risk of osteoporosis when compared with other populations.

The biggest value of multicentre studies is that it increases what is called the generalizability of the trial to other populations. The methodological problem inherited with multicentre studies is that each of us does things a little differently, and we need to be much more rigorous in our control as to how the trial is conducted.

13

Pharmacology of the luteinizing hormone-releasing hormone (LHRH) analogue, Zoladex*

B.J.A. Furr

INTRODUCTION

It is well established that androgens stimulate the growth of a majority of prostate cancers, and oestrogens enhance the growth of many breast cancers. A variety of approaches have been adopted to induce androgen or oestrogen withdrawal from the tumour cell in order to prevent prostate and breast tumour progression. Anti-oestrogens such as Nolvadex[1*] and anti-androgens such as cyproterone acetate[2], flutamide[3], nilutamide[4] and Casodex[5*], compete with the relevant stimulatory hormone to bind to a cytosolic receptor protein, but have little or no intrinsic activity as oestrogens or androgens, respectively.

A knowledge of the processes that regulate gonadal steroid synthesis has led to further approaches to tumour therapy. Administration of oestrogens to men with prostate cancer inhibits gonadotrophin secretion from the pituitary gland, leading to a form of medical castration[6]. However, the clinical benefits seen in prostate cancer patients may be counterbalanced by serious cardiovascular complications[7].

*Zoladex, Nolvadex and Casodex are trade names, the property of Imperial Chemical Industries PLC

147

Recently, the availability of potent analogues of luteinizing hormone-releasing hormone (LHRH) has led to a selective effect on pituitary gonadotrophin release that produces a form of medical castration. The side-effects are markedly less than those associated with the administration of oestrogens and indeed the only side-effects reported are those which might be predicted from a medical castration. Zoladex (goserelin, D-Ser (Bu^t)^6, Azgly^{10}-LHRH; Figure 1), is a potent LHRH analogue, which can be used for the treatment of hormone-responsive disease[8]. This paper describes pharmacological studies with Zoladex, attempts to explain its mode of action and reports on an innovative depot formulation, which allows the drug to be released continuously over at least 28 days.

Pyro - Glu - His - Trp - Ser - Tyr - Gly - Leu - Arg - Pro - Gly - NH$_2$

LH - RH

Pyro - Glu - His - Trp - Ser - Tyr - |D - Ser (Bu^t)| - Leu - Arg - Pro - |Azgly NH$_2$|

ZOLADEX (ICI 118,630 D - SER (Bu ^{t})^6 AzGly^{10} - LH - RH)

Figure 1   Structures of LHRH and Zoladex

PHARMACOLOGICAL STUDIES WITH AQUEOUS SOLUTIONS OF AN LHRH AGONIST – ZOLADEX

Zoladex is an LHRH agonist (LHRH–A) and when given acutely, will induce release of follicle-stimulating hormone (FSH) and luteinizing hormone (LH) secretion. In the rat, a single intramusclar injection of 5 μg Zoladex elicits a supraphysiological release of LH (Figure 2). In this respect it is at least 100 times as potent as LHRH[9].

Zoladex will also initiate LH release and ovulation in androgen-sterilized constant oestrus rats (Table 1). When given by the intramuscular (i.m.), subcutaneous (s.c.) or intravenous (i.v.), routes, Zoladex is at least 100 times as potent as LHRH. It should be emphasized, however, that it is far less effective when given intravaginally, orally (p.o.) or intranasally, and in the latter case absorption is both low and variable.

148

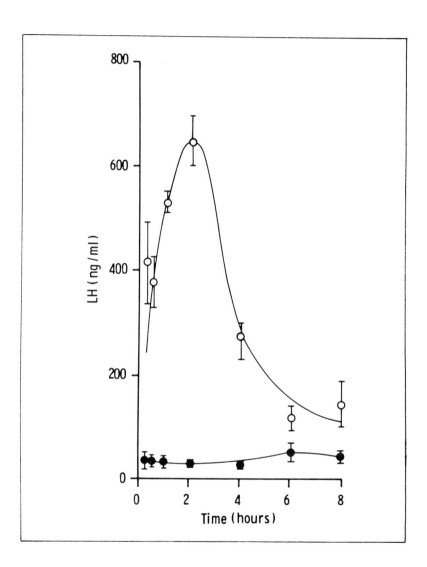

Figure 2 Plasma LH concentrations in mature virgin female rats given a single i.m. injection of 5 μg Zoladex at time O (open circles). The closed circles are the values for saline-treated controls. The points indicated are the mean values for 5 animals with the standard error of the mean

Table 1 Induction of ovulation with Zoladex given intraveneously, orally, intravaginally or intranasally in androgen-sterilized, constant oestrus rats

Route	Dose µg	Number ovulating/ number treated	Response %
Intravenous	0.005	9/9	100
	0.0031	10/18	55.6
	0.0016	5/21	23.8
	0.0008	0/12	0
Oral	25	3/3	100
	10	5/6	83.3
	5	5/12	41.7
	2.5	2/6	33
Intravaginal	25	2/3	67
	10	0/3	0
Intranasal	1	2/5	40

The high potency of Zoladex is partly due to its enhanced affinity for the pituitary LHRH receptor (Figure 3), which leads to around a 10-fold greater potency compared with LHRH, in releasing LH from pituitary cells in culture (Figure 4). The high potency *in vivo* is also due to a longer elimination half-life: in man, the half-life of Zoladex is more than 4 hours, compared with less than 10 minutes for LHRH[10].

When given chronically, Zoladex induces inhibition of gonadal steroid secretion and produces a castration-like state in rats, dogs and primates[8,11,12]. At first sight, this is unexpected and has therefore been inappropriately described as the paradoxical effect of LHRH agonists. An explanation for this observation is clearly required.

MODE OF ACTION OF LHRH AGONISTS

Normally, LHRH is released from the hypothalamus as a series of small pulses, at approximately 90 minute intervals[13,14]. The LHRH travels via the hypothalamic–pituitary portal system to the pituitary gland where it binds to LHRH receptors present on the cell surface. Receptors occupied

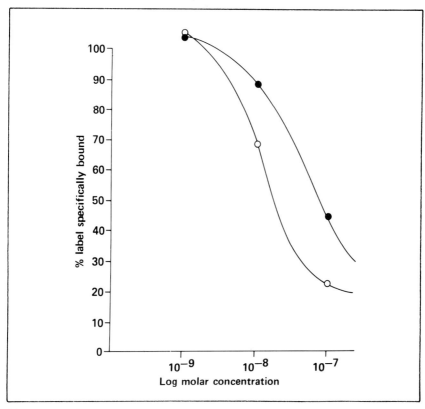

Figure 3 Relative potencies of Zoladex (O) and LHRH (●) in causing displacement of
^{125}I-D-Leu^6-proethylamide^9-LHRH from a rat pituitary membrane receptor preparation

by LHRH aggregate into clumps, 'coated pits' are formed and the
receptor–ligand complex is internalised, thus disappearing from the cell
surface. There is usually an excess of LHRH receptors present on the
pituitary cell and receptor resynthesis occurs. This process allows an
orderly and systematic secretion of LH. When an LHRH agonist is first
given at a relatively high dosage, the majority of LHRH receptors are
occupied and subsequently internalised. This leads to supraphysiological
LH secretion and an intitial stimulation of gonadal function. However,
the marked loss of LH receptors and the failure of receptor replenishment
due to the continuing presence of LHRH–A leads to a pituitary cell
which has few receptors, and is, therefore, unable to respond to
LHRH–A. Consequently, LH secretion is markedly reduced, resulting in

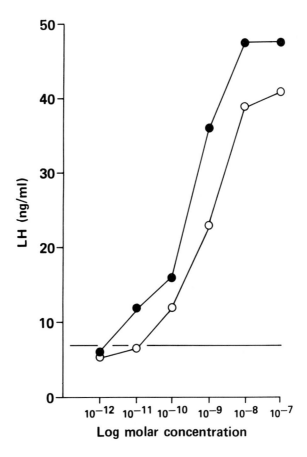

Figure 4 Release of LH from dispersed rat pituitary cells into the culture medium after 4 hours incubation in response to increasing concentration of Zoladex (●) and LHRH (O). Control values shown by the horizontal line indicate the release rate in the absence of LHRH or LHRH agonist

gonadal atrophy, a reduction in steroid secretion and the regression of hormone-responsive tissues including mammary and prostate tumours.

This phenomenon had long been recognised and termed either tachyphylaxis or tissue desensitization, but is now described as receptor down-regulation. It is clearly a predictable, non-paradoxical effect of chronic therapy with LHRH agonists. Usually tachyphylaxis is regarded as a serious disadvantage in a drug therapy. Here, for the first time, advantage is taken of this phenomenon to produce an effective therapy.

DEVELOPMENT AND PROPERTIES OF A DEPOT
FORMULATION OF ZOLADEX

Although early preclinical studies clearly demonstrate the effectiveness of daily s.c. injections in inducing regression of sex hormone-responsive tumours[11], it was felt that this would limit clinical acceptability and reduce patient compliance with therapy. Several formulations were considered, but the majority were rejected because of concerns about reliability of drug delivery or convenience. Adminstration of Zoladex by vaginal pessaries limited treatment to women, and absorption was low and variable. Similarly, in our experience, absorption of the drug after nasal adminstration was also low and unacceptably variable. Furthermore, nasal application had to be made several times daily to achieve the desired biological effect, which again raised concerns about the likelihood of compliance. Others have found nasal spray formulations to be acceptable, but compliance is recognized as a problem[15].

The target selected for a drug delivery system for Zoladex was the development of a biodegradable, sustained-release formulation that would deliver the drug over a period of at least 28 days. Efforts were concentrated on poly(d,1-lactide) and poly(d,1,lactide-*co*-glycolide) since these have been used for the sustained delivery of low molecular weight compounds such as steroids[16], narcotic antagonists[17] and antimalarial drugs[18]. Moreover, since these polymers have been evaluated as biodegradable surgical sutures and prostheses, it is known that they are both pharmaceutically and toxicologically acceptable. This work culminated in the development of a depot based on a 50:50 poly(d,1-lactide-*co*-glycolide) polymer throughout which the drug is homogeneously dispersed. The depot is in the form of a rod approximately 1 mm in diameter and 3–6 mm in length containing 500–1000 µg Zoladex. Following administration of a single depot containing 500 µg Zoladex, oestrogen secretion, assessed by vaginal smear inspection, is suppressed in adult female rats for 33 days (Figure 5).

Although the primary objective was to produce a formulation of the drug that was more convenient to administer and that would secure improved compliance, the depot formulation also appears to have improved efficacy. This was demonstrated in rats that were given a single s.c. bolus dose of 50 µg Zoladex for 6 weeks or, alternatively, at the start of the experiment and at 4 weeks, a single s.c. depot, calculated to release

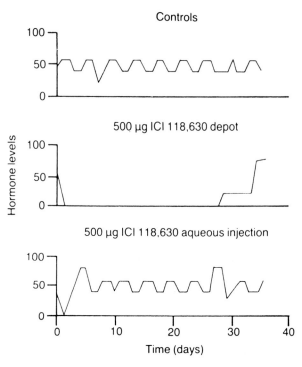

Figure 5 Effect of a single s.c. injection of 500 μg Zoladex (ICI 118,630) either as a depot formulation or as an aqueous injection in 1% hydroxymethylcellulose on ovarian activity in adult female rats. Control data are shown in the upper panel for comparison

a dose of Zoladex equivalent to 50 μg daily. Rats were killed at various times after the final treatment and serum LH was determined by radioimmunoassay in blood collected from the dorsal aorta (Figure 6).

As expected, the bolus dose of Zoladex elicited a massive secretion of LH in rats pretreated with saline. In spite of pretreatment for 6 weeks with 50 μg Zoladex daily, the bolus dose of the drug still caused a substantial release of LH, although a clear degree of desensitization of the pituitary gland occurred. In contrast, there was negligible LH secretion in response to the bolus injection in rats pretreated with Zoladex depot, indicating an improved level of pituitary desensitization by this formulation. Similarly, in the male monkey, *Maccaca nemestrina*, the depot formulation of Zoladex induces a fall in plasma testosterone into the castrate range, whereas daily s.c. injections are relatively ineffective. (It

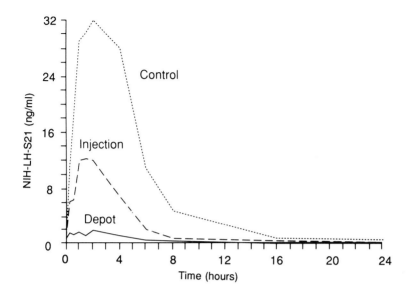

Figure 6 Effect of a 50 μg s.c. bolus dose of Zoladex on LH release in mature male rats given either saline or 50 μg Zoladex daily or a single s.c. depot containing Zoladex calculated to release approximately 50 μg daily at the start of the experiment and at day 28. The bolus dose of 50 μg Zoladex was injected 6 weeks after the start of the experiment and serum LH was measured by radioimmunoassay at the times shown

should be noted that recovery of testicular function occurred around 40 days after the final depot was administered.) This advantage of depot Zoladex has also been observed in the clinic where incomplete pituitary desensitization is seen in some patients given daily s.c. injections of the drug, in contrast to complete pituitary desensitization in those given Zoladex depot[19].

EFFECTS OF DEPOT ZOLADEX IN ANIMALS BEARING SEX HORMONE-RESPONSIVE TUMOURS

The androgen responsive, Dunning R3327H, transplantable rat, prostate tumour[20] was used in several studies to determine the efficacy of Zoladex depot adminstration. Single s.c. depots containing 1 mg Zoladex given every 28 days to rats bearing Dunning R3327H prostate tumours, implanted on each flank, produced a marked inhibition of tumour growth, similar to that seen in surgically castrated rats (Figure 7). Twenty-one days after the eighth depot was given, the rats were killed and the weights of the sex organs assessed and serum hormone concentrations measured by radioimmunoassay. Testes weights were about 10% of those of control rats of a similar age and weight, and showed atrophic histological changes; ventral prostate gland and seminal vesicle weights were identical to those in the surgically castrated group and, histologically, were also completely atrophic. Serum LH and testosterone were undetectable in the group given Zoladex depot and serum FSH level was decreased by 60–70%.

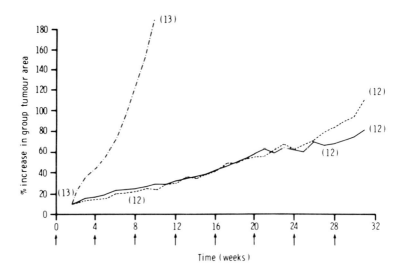

Figure 7 Growth of Dunning R3327H androgen-responsive prostate tumours in male rats, which were either surgically castrated (—) or given a single s.c. depot without Zoladex (·--·) or containing 1 mg Zoladex (----) at 28 day intervals on eight occasions as shown by the arrows. The values are expressed as percent increase in mean tumour area

A comparison was made of the efficacy of surgical castration, depot Zoladex, a new peripherally-selective anti-androgen, ICI 176,334 (Casodex)[5] and the combination, in the treatment of Dunning R3327H prostate tumours (Figure 8). All treatments produced a significant

Estimated Mean Tumour Areas With Standard Errors (Geometric)

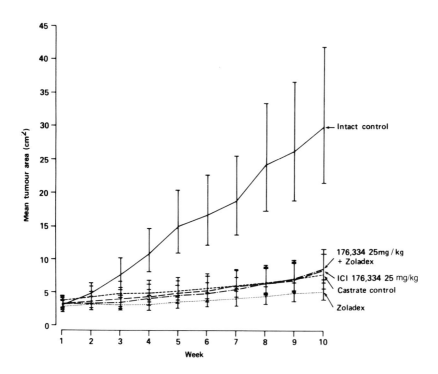

Figure 8 Effect of surgical castration, depot Zoladex given s.c. every 28 days, ICI 176,334 (novel peripherally-selective antiandrogen) given p.o. daily and the combination of the two drugs on growth of the Dunning R3327H prostate tumour. Data from intact control animals are shown for comparison. The results show the mean tumour area ± SEM

reduction in tumour growth compared to control animals, but none of the treatments was any more effective than another. Since the rat does not secrete significant quantities of adrenal androgens, these data cannot be taken to disprove the total androgen withdrawal hypothesis advanced by Labrie and colleagues[21].

Zoladex depot has also proved to be highly effective against dimethylbenzanthracene-induced rat mammary tumours. Adminstration of single s.c. depots containing 500 µg Zoladex every 28 days produced inhibition of oestrogen secretion, disappearance of cornified cells from vaginal smears and frequently, complete tumour regression[11]. When given at days 30, 58 and 86 after adminstration of the carcinogen, single depots containing 500 µg Zoladex delayed the appearance of tumours for a period of around 100 days, i.e. the expected duration of action of such a treatment regimen[11].

When given at 28 day intervals, starting on day 30 after administration of the carcinogen, single s.c. depots of Zoladex caused a more profound inhibition of tumour appearance and only nine out of 27 rats had mammary tumours at the end of the study on day 450[11]. The tumours that remained did not regress following ovariectomy, and were therefore classified as non-hormone responsive. It is concluded from this study (which approximates the adjuvant therapy setting) that Zoladex may be of benefit as a treatment for primary breast cancer after mastectomy in premenopausal women.

No side-effects were observed in any of these studies, and there was no lesion at any injection site.

CONCLUSION

Zoladex in common with other potent LHRH agonistic analogues when given chronically at relatively high doses, causes a predictable pituitary desensitization and consequently an inhibition of pituitary gonadotrophin secretion. This in turn leads to gonadal and accessory sex organ atrophy.

The biodegradable, biocompatible Zoladex depot which releases the drug continuously over at least 28 days, is both more convenient to administer and more efficacious in a number of test systems than are daily s.c. injections. In particular, it is highly effective at inducing regression of sex hormone-responsive prostate and mammary tumours. The pharmacological profile of Zoladex depot, its excellent tolerance and its convenience of adminstration make it an effective alternative to surgery for treatment of sex hormone-responsive tumours in men and women, and in a number of other disorders dependent upon or modified by gonadal sex steroids.

ACKNOWLEDGEMENTS

NIAMDD, Professor L.E. Reichert and G.D. Niswender for reagents for FSH, LH and prolactin radioimmunoassays. The US National Prostate Cancer Agency for supplies of rats bearing Dunning R3327H tumours. The many colleagues in ICI Pharmaceuticals Research Department, who have made this development possible, particularly A.S. Dutta, F.G. Hutchinson and B.E. Valcaccia. This paper originally appeared in *Hormone Research* (1989) published by S. Karger AG, Basel.

REFERENCES

1. Furr, B.J.A. and Jordan, V.C. (1984). The pharmacology and clinical uses of tamoxifen. *Pharmacol. Ther.*, **25**, 127–205

2. Neumann, F. (1987). Pharmacology and clinical uses of cyproterone acetate. In Furr, B.J.A. and Wakeling, A.E. (eds.). *Pharmacology and Clinical Uses of Inhibitors of Hormone Secretion and Action*, pp. 132–59. (London: Balliere Tindall)

3. Neri, R. and Kassem, N. (1987). Pharmacology and clinical uses of flutamide. In Furr, B.J.A. and Wakeling, A.E. (eds.). *Pharmacology and Clinical Uses of Inhibitors of Hormone Secretion and Action*, pp. 160–9. (London: Balliere Tindall)

4. Moguilewsky, M., Fiet, J., Tournemine, G. and Raynaud, J-P. (1986). Pharmacology of an anti-androgen, Anandron, used as an adjuvant therapy in the treatment of prostate cancer. *J. Steroid. Biochem.*, **24**, 139–46

5. Furr, B.J.A., Valaccia, B., Curry, B., Woodburn, J.R., Chesterson, G. and Tucker, H. (1987). ICI 176,334: a novel non-steroidal, peripherally selective anti-androgen. *J. Endocrinol.*, **113**, R7–R9

6. Robinson, M.R.G. (1982). Carcinoma of the prostate: hormonal therapy. In Furr, B.J.A. (ed.). *Clinics in oncology*, vol. 1, pp. 233–43. (London: Saunders)

7. Veterans Adminstration Cooperative Urological Research Group. (1967). Treatment and survival of patients with cancer of the prostate. *Surg. Gynecol. Obstet.*, **124**, 1011–17

8. Furr, B.J.A. (1987). Treatment of hormone-responsive rat mammary and prostate tumours with Zoladex depot. In Klijn, J.G.M., Paridaens, R. and Foekens, J.A. (eds.). *Hormonal Manipulation of Cancer: Peptides, Growth Factors and New (Anti) Steroidal Agents*. Monograph Series of the European Organisation for Research on Treatment of Cancer (EORTC), vol. 18,

pp. 213–23. (New York: Raven Press)

9. Maynard, P.V. and Nicholson, R.I. (1979). Biological effects of high dose levels of a series of new LHRH analogues in intact female rats. *Br. J. Cancer*, **39**, 274–9

10. Swaisland, A.J., Adam, H.K., Barker, Y., Holmes, B. and Hutchinson, F.G. (1988). Tailored release profiles for Zoladex using biodegradable polymers. *Pharm. Weekbl.*, **10**, 57

11. Furr, B.J.A. and Nicholson, R.I. (1982). Use of analogues of luteinising hormone-releasing hormone-releasing hormone for the treatment of cancer. *J. Reprod. Fertil.*, **64**, 529–39

12. Furr, B.J.A. and Hutchinson, F.G. (1985). Biodegradable sustained release formulation of the LHRH analogue Zoladex for the treatment of hormone-responsive tumours. In Schroeder, F.H. and Richards, B. (eds.). EORTC Genitourinary Group Monograph 2, Part A. *Therapeutic Principles in Metastatic Prostatic Cancer*. Progress in Clinical and Biochemical Research, vol. 185A, pp. 143–53. (New York: Liss)

13. Nankin, H.R. and Troen, R. (1971). Repetitive luteinising hormone elevations in serum of normal men. *J. Clin. Endocrinol. Metab.*, **33**, 558–60

14. Santen, R.J. and Bardin, C.W. (1973). Episodic luteinising hormone secretion in man. *J. Clin. Invest.*, **52**, 2617–28

15. Rajfer, J., Handelsman, D.J., Crum, A., Steiner, B., Peterson, M. and Swerdloff, R.S. (1986). Comparison of the efficacy of subcutaneous and nasal spray buserelin treatment in suppression of testicular steroidogenesis in men with prostate cancer. *Fertil. Steril.*, **46**, 104–10

16. Beck, L.R., Cowsar, D.R., Lewis, D.H., Cosgrove, J.R., Riddle, C.T., Lowry, S.L. and Epperly, T. (1979). A new long-acting injectable microcapsule system for the adminstration of progesterone. *Fertil. Steril.*, **31**, 545–51

17. Schwope, A.D., Wise, D.L. and Howed, J.F. (1975). Lactic/glycolic acid polymers as narcotic antagonist delivery systems. *Life Sci.*, 1877–85

18. Wise, D.L., McCormick, G.J., Willet, G.P. and Anderson, L.C. (1976). Sustained release of an antimalarial drug using copolymer of glycolic/lactic acid. *Life Sci.*, 867–73

19. Grant, J.B.F., Ahmed, S.R., Shalet, S.M., Costello, C.B., Howell, A. and Blacklock, N.J. (1986). Testosterone and gonadotrophin profiles in patients on daily or monthly LHRH analogue (Zoladex) compared with orchidectomy. *Br. J. Urol.*, **58**, 539–44

20. Smolev, J.K., Heston, W.D.W., Scott, W.W. and Coffey, D.S. (1977). Characterization of the Dunning R3327H prostatic adenocarcinoma: an appropriate animal model for prostatic cancer. *Cancer. Treat. Rep.*, **61**, 273–87

21. Labrie, F., Dupont, A. and Belanger, A. (1985). Complete androgen blockade for the treatment of prostate cancer. In De Vita, V.T. Jr, Hellman, S. and Rosenberg, S.A. (eds.). *Important Advances in Oncology*, pp. 193–217. (Philadelphia: Lippincott)

DISCUSSION

Prof. Donnez

What would suppress the flare-up effect we observe when we start this kind of treatment?

Dr Furr

I am not sure what is meant by 'flare-up' in the female context. In the trials we have looked at we do not get a disease flare at the start of the treatment in the woman.

Prof. Donnez

Could combining an agonist with an antagonist at the commencement of treatment be a good strategy?

Dr Furr

I would not have thought so because the antagonist has a much shorter duration of action and it will compromise the down-regulation effect that we see with the agonist. There may be some value in total oestrogen withdrawal if there is value in total androgen withdrawal, which is still in dispute, and it may be worth giving a steroid antagonist like Nolvadex with the LHRH agonist Zoladex in patients with breast cancer.

But in endometriosis the oestrogen withdrawal that is achieved is sufficient to cause responses in the majority of patients.

Dr Wheeler

Could Dr Furr comment perhaps on the difference in the loading mechanism between an implant such as Zoladex and polyglycolic microcapsules which some other companies are starting to investigate for delivery of peptide hormones?

Dr Furr

We can argue about what is a microcapsule. I think that they are not microcapsules but microspheres and that they are just crushed up versions of an LHRH agonist in powdered form, a small round form.

A true microcapsule to me, and the definition to a pharmaceutical person, is that the drug is encapsulated within the polymer. Those do not appear to be of that type.

Dr Wheeler

What worries me is that the 'microspheres' have a great variability compared to a standardized implant and it will be trickier for them to have a good standardized absorption curve as compared with a standard implant.

Dr Furr

They certainly have a much larger surface area and it will be more difficult, but the actual release mechanism, which is a diffusion followed by a degradation, would be similar.

14

Future management of endometriosis – GnRH analogues

R.W. Shaw

INTRODUCTION

The continuing growth and development of endometriotic tissue depends upon oestrogen. This condition is prevalent in the reproductive years with a peak incidence between 30 and 45 years of age, and it is still not established whether mild endometriosis is an early manifestation of progressive disease in the majority of individuals. The treatment chosen depends upon the extent, site and symptoms of the disease, the patient's age and her desire for future pregnancy. Surgical treatment is tailored to the individual needs of the patient and may be either conservative, aimed at normalizing and maintaining the genital tract for future reproductive use, or radical which may include complete pelvic clearance as a means of eliminating the disease.

Medical treatment has also been utilized and includes pseudopregnancy regimes, continuous oral contraceptive therapy, progestagens alone, danazol or gestrinone. Many of these regimes are effective therapies, but side-effects accompanying their use can be severe resulting in certain patients discontinuing treatment. New and more effective therapies have therefore been sought, and currently the possibility of selectively suppressing the ovarian secretion of steroids by repeated administration of GnRH analogues is under intensive investigation.

GnRH ANALOGUES

Competitive exposure of the pituitary gonadotrophe cells to potent GnRH agonistic analogues induces endocrine changes with resultant hypogonadotrophic hypogonadism. Mechanisms of action by which GnRH agonists achieve this state are discussed in detail in the preceding chapter. All of the GnRH agonists currently undergoing clinical trials are extremely potent compared with the native GnRH. Whilst it may be desirable to try to achieve graded desensitization of the hypothalamic–pituitary–ovarian axis, in practice this is extremely difficult. The differences between the potencies of the various GnRH agonistic analogues in terms of their endocrine effects thus become of little relevance. Perhaps of more paramount importance is the development of adequate and reliable delivery systems. GnRH agonists are available in a number of formulations. For conditions which require short-term adminstration of GnRH analogues, daily subcutaneous formulations may be suitable. However, in conditions such as endometriosis requiring prolonged treatment and perhaps repetitive adminstration regimes, a slow-release depot formulation may offer certain advantages. Intranasal delivery systems have also been widely used in prolonged treatment regimes because of simplicity of patient use. However, variation in absorption rates can be quite marked related to the molecular size and hydrophilic/lipophilic characteristics of the peptide and its stability. In addition, the multiple daily adminstration necessary with such formulations can have disadvantages.

Depot formulations of with life expectancy of 1 or 3 months thus offer many attractions. A number of hydrophobic polymers and hydrogels are available which are biodegradable and would make an acceptable formulation. The other advantage of a sustained release formulation is the implicit ability to overcome patient non-compliance.

The structures of some GnRH agonists currently under investigation in the treatment of endometriosis are listed in Table 1.

STUDIES OF GnRH ANALOGUES IN THE TREATMENT OF ENDOMETRIOSIS

Meldrum and colleagues first reported the use of a GnRH analogue in

five women with endometriosis who received D-Trp⁶PRO⁹ Net LHRH
as a daily subcutaneous injection for a period of 1 month[1]. Endocrine
response was compared with women who had undergone
oophorectomy. In the month of treatment serum levels of FSH decreased
below basal levels and LH levels rose slightly above baseline. In four out
of the five patients oestradiol concentrations were within the castrate
range. The first definitive attempts to treat endometriosis for a long
period of time were reported by Shaw and colleagues[2]. In this study six
patients were treated for 6 months with the GnRH analogue D-SER-
tBu⁶PRO⁹ Net LHRH (buserelin). Five subjects received 200 ug
intranasally three times daily and the sixth patient a single daily dose of
400 ug intranasally. Five patients completed the 6 months of treatment
and at repeat laparoscopy resolution of endometriotic lesions was
observed. During treatment ovulation was suppressed and oestradiol
levels were well below those seen in the earlier follicular phase of the
cycle, and some patients complained of experiencing hot flushes. The
patient who received a daily dose of 400 ug had a more advanced stage of
the disease and ceased treatment after 3 months due to increasing
enlargement of her endometrioma and failure to control symptoms. In
1984 Lemay and colleagues published the results on a further series of 10
patients receiving D-SER-tBu⁶PRO⁹ Net LHRH (buserelin) between
25 and 31 weeks, either as twice daily subcutaneous injections or 400 ug
intranasally three times daily[3]. Again, a dramatic reduction in endo-

Table 1 Amino acid sequence of native GnRH and some of its agonistic
analogues used in treatment of endometriosis

	1	2	3	4	5	(6)	7	8	9	(10)
GnRH	p-GLU – HIS – TRP – SER – TYR – GLY – LEU – ARG – PRO – GLY–NH₂								
Buserelin						D-Ser(Buᵗ)			PRO-NET –	
Leuprolide						D-Leu			PRO-NET –	
Histrelin						D-His(1mBel)			PRO-NET –	
Nafarelin						(D-Nal)²				
Tryptoretin						(D-Trp)				
Goserelin						D-Ser(Buᵗ)			Az-Gly	

metriotic deposits was observed as assessed at repeat laparoscopy, but at these higher doses of the analogue side-effects of oestrogen deficiency, in particular hot flushes and dryness of the vagina, were reported in many subjects.

These pilot investigations indicated GnRH analogues were a safe and effective treatment for endometriosis. Further uncontrolled studies have since been published in larger series of patients, evaluating different analogues and varying dose regimes[4-6].

STRATEGY IN THE TREATMENT OF ENDOMETRIOSIS

The strategy in the treatment of endometriosis is as outlined in Figure 1. It is believed that to achieve relief of symptoms and to arrest spread, and induce regression of endometriotic deposits, then a situation of hypo-oestrogenism and suppression of menstruation are beneficial. To evaluate GnRH analogues in this respect it is advantageous to compare them in terms of efficacy and patient tolerance with other established medical treatments, in particular, against the most widely used and effective treatment currently available – danazol. Such comparative studies have been initiated and the results of these are now beginning to be reported in the literature.

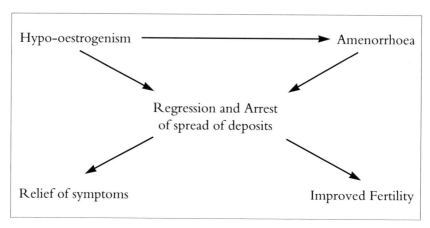

Figure 1 Strategy in the treatment of endometriosis

Development of hypo-oestrogenism

The adminstration of GnRH analogue therapy during the early follicular phase of the cycle results in an initial agonistic-induced surge of gonadotrophins with a sustained and marked increase of LH and FSH persisting over a period of some days. Within a few days, however, pituitary desensitization occurs, FSH levels return to pretreatment basal levels by the fourth or fifth day of adminstration of GnRH agonists and LH basal levels are achieved within 7–10 days. Thereafter LH and FSH remain at or below baseline early follicular phase levels. The initial agonistic surge of gonadotrophins induces an increase in serum oestradiol levels from stimulated follicule maturation. Again, within 3–4 days oestrogen levels begin to fall and have fallen below early follicular phase values by the seventh day of administration, and have usually fallen further to within the postmenopausal range by the end of the first therapy at which they remain throughout continued treatment. These initial acute gonadotrophin and ovarian steroid changes are demonstrated in Figure 2 in a group of subjects receiving a single 3.6 mg depot formulation of D-Ser(Bu^t)^6-AzaGly^{10} LHRH (Zoladex).

The degree of ovarian suppression achieved was evaluated using a number of different analogues and compared with danazol. The three analogues studied were D (Nal$_2$)^6 LHRH (nafarelin), buserelin and goserelin. All three analogues achieved suppression within the first month of therapy to levels comparable to the early follicular phase and in many subjects to within the postmenopausal range, with the suppression being maintained throughout the remainder of the 6 months of therapy. The degree of suppression achieved with the three analogues was greater than that produced in patients receiving danazol at a dose of 600 mg daily. The depot GnRH analogue preparation of goserelin appeared to achieve a more consistent and profound hypo-oestrogen in effect than the two intranasal preparations nafarelin and buserelin in this study and at the doses studied (Figure 3).

Induction of amenorrhoea

One presumed important objective in the treatment of patients with endometriosis is to produce a prolonged period of absent endometrial shedding and menstrual bleedings. Periods of continual or intermittent

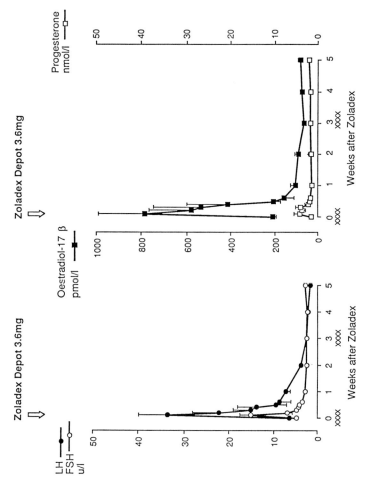

Figure 2 The initial acute agonistic induced changes in serum LH, FSH, oestradiol-17β and progesterone in a group of nine regularly menstruating women receiving a single 3.6 mg depot injection of the GnRH analogue goserelin (D-Ser(Bu^t)^6 – Aza Gly LHRH – Zoladex, ICI Pharmaceuticals)

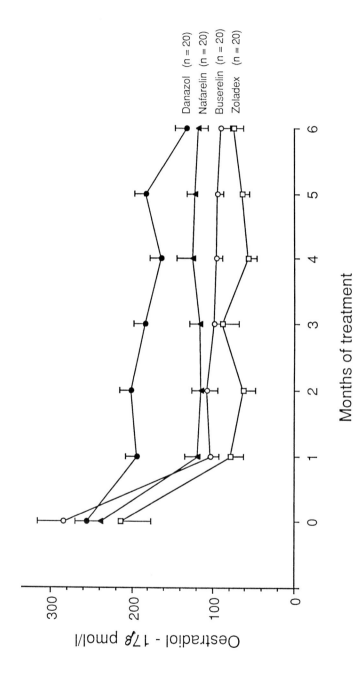

Figure 3 Comparative degrees of hypo–oestrogenism achieved during 6-months therapy with the GnRH analogues nafarelin 200 μg bd. intranasally, buserelin 300 μg t.d.s. intranasally, 3.6 mg depot Zoladex monthly and danazol 200 mg t.d.s.

bleeding within the endometriotic deposits is thought to be one factor in the induction of local tissue reaction and adhesion formation. Inhibition of such cyclical bleeding is necessary to increase the speed at which resolution and healing of such deposits may occur. The percentage of patients on a monthly basis in whom induction of amenorrhoea was achieved was evaluated in groups of patients receiving either danazol, goserelin, nafarelin or buserelin during 6 months of therapy (Table 2). Complete amenorrhoea was achieved in a higher proportion of patients receiving danazol than either of the three GnRH analogues only in the first month of therapy. This is because an oestrogen withdrawal bleed occurs in the majority of patients receiving a GnRH analogue between 14 and 22 days after commencement of the treatment when started during the menstrual phase of the cycle. In the second month of treatment with GnRH analogues, however, few patients had bleeding episodes indicating the attainment of adequate hypo-oestrogenism following pituitary desensitization. The depot preparation goserelin which induces a more profound degree of hypo-oestrogenism (as demonstrated previously in Figure 3) resulted in a higher percentage of subjects with complete amenorrhoea being maintained throughout treatment. However, there was no direct correlation between circulating oestradiol-17β levels and episodes of menstrual bleeding.

The return of the first spontaneous menstrual period upon ceasing therapy is comparable on all treatments (Table 2). However, with the depot preparation goserelin the time to first menstruation was calculated as from 28 days following adminstration of the last implant – the presumed normal lifespan of the implant – whilst for danazol, naferelin and buserelin it was calculated from the last day of the administration of the drug. It is apparent, therefore, that GnRH analogues compare favourably with danazol in their ability to induce amenorrhoea as a treatment criteria for endometriosis.

The resolution of endometrial deposits

In our study performed on 62 patients entered into an open, randomized comparative trial of buserelin 400 ug t.d.s. intranasally and danazol 200 mg t.d.s., the extent of endometriosis was staged according to the revised American Fertility Society (rAFS) classification, both at the commencement

Table 2 Percentage (%) of patients with amenorrhoea during 6 months treatment for endometriosis with either danazol, nafarelin, goserelin or buserelin

Month of treatment	Danazol 200 mg tds n = 20	Nafarelin 200 μg bd n = 20	Goserelin 3.6 mg monthly n = 40	Buserelin 300 μg tds n = 20
1	35	10	15	5
2	51	80	97.5	85
3	80	85	97.5	80
4	90	80	97.5	90
5	90	85	97.5	95
6	85	90	97.5	95
Return to first menses (Days)	30–56	28–58	31–75	27–64

of treatment and at the end of the 6 months treatment course.

This study showed that in 82% of patients who received buserelin, no visible endometriotic deposits were found at the end of 6 months treatment. The comparable figure in patients receiving danazol was 72%[7]. This represented a highly significant improvement in the staging of the disease but no significant difference between the two treatment modalities. The percentage of patients having no residual deposits at repeat laparoscopy was highest in patients who initially had mild disease, whether treated with the GnRH analogue or danazol. Comparable responses from the two treatments were seen in a reduction of AFS scores in moderate disease, but because of smaller numbers of patients with severe disease it is uncertain whether one treatment is superior to another (Figure 4). Recently a multicentre study comparing two doses of the GnRH agonist nafarelin against danazol in a placebo-controlled double-blind study reported comparable findings[8].

These comparative trials indicate that GnRH agonists are as effective as danazol in inducing suppression and resolution of endometriotic deposits. It is apparent from these studies, however, that peritoneal deposits respond far more effectively than ovarian deposits and that deep-seated ovarian disease, particularly endometriomas in excess of 3 cm diameter, respond poorly.

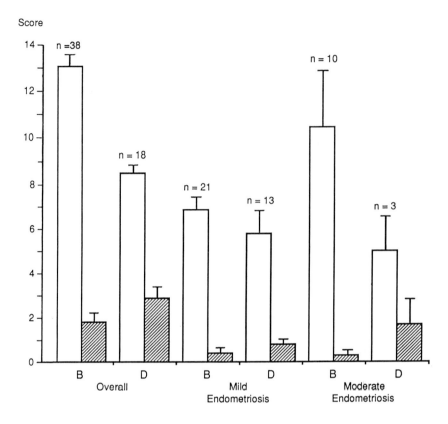

Score

Figure 4 Changes in AFS point scores for endometriotic deposits (excluding adhesion contribution) in randomized patients to B – buserelin 400 µg t.d.s. intranasally or D – danazol 400–800 mg daily with mild or moderate endometriosis. Hatched column indicates reduction following 6 months treatment

Relief of symptoms

Some of the less common symptoms in patients with endometriosis are dependent upon the site of the deposits. However, symptoms of dysmenorrhoea, dyspareunia and pelvic pain are commonly found in patients proven to have endometriosis. These symptoms can be readily categorized on a points scale for severity; the degree of severity does not correlate with AFS point score. The comparative trials[7,8] have reported a good response in terms of relief of these common symptoms during treatment with GnRH agonists, and the results compare favourably with those achieved in patients receiving danazol. It is perhaps not surprising that dysmenorrhoea is the symptom which is most rapidly relieved as suppression of menstruation is induced. Deep dyspareunia is improved after 1 month of therapy and improvement continues to increase with the increasing duration of therapy. Pelvic pain is a more diffuse symptom, perhaps a reflection of more deep-seated endometriotic disease, and takes longer to become completely relieved.

In the majority of women if amenorrhoea is induced there appears to be little difference between danazol and GnRH analogues in terms of achieving relief of symptoms at the end of 6 months of therapy.

RECURRENCE OF ENDOMETRIOSIS

Data from our initial uncontrolled studies indicated that patients who received GnRH agonists with apparently good initial response, in some instances developed proven recurrence of the disease within 6–12 months of ceasing therapy and return to normal menstrual cycle. In patients entered into our randomized comparative trial of buserelin against danazol[7], laparoscopy confirmed recurrence in six of the 39 patients treated with buserelin and in three of the 18 patients treated with danazol, during the initial 12 month follow-up period. Recurrence was more likely to occur in patients with moderate or severe disease. In a number of subjects they were monitored with serial measurements of serum CA-125 levels and circulating levels of CA-125 in excess of 35 u/ml were suggestive of recurrence[9]. Six out of nine patients with CA-125 above 35 u/ml had proven recurrence whereas only three out of 45 patients with levels below 35 u/ml developed symptomatic recurrence. However, only patients with recurrent symptoms had a further repeat laparoscopy amongst this group of subjects who had all previously been symptomatic. It is possible, therefore, that some other patients who were currently asymptomatic would have some laparoscopic evidence of recurrence.

SIDE-EFFECTS OF GnRH ANALOGUES

It would be surprising if the high degree of hypo-oestrogenism induced by GnRH agonists did not produce some symptoms of oestrogen deficiency in patients on long-term therapy for endometriosis. The majority of subjects can be expected to experience hot flushes by the second and third months of treatment which may be both frequent and severe in some individuals. Headaches and vaginal dryness are more frequently found in patients receiving GnRH analogues than danazol (see Table 3). This symptom profile has to be compared against the androgenic and systemic side-effects commonly experienced in patients on danazol (see Table 3).

Table 3 Pretreatment symptoms (%) and side-effects induced during 6 months therapy with danazol 400–800 mg daily ($n = 40$) or Zoladex depot 3.6 mg monthly ($n = 32$)

	Danazol group (n = 40)				Zoladex group (n = 32)			
	Pre-treatment	*1mth*	*3mth*	*6mth*	*Pre-treatment*	*1mth*	*3mth*	*6mth*
Hot flushes	2.5	5.0	15.0	27.5	3.0	71.8	92.1	90.5
Sweats	5.0	5.0	10.0	15.0	4.8	46.2	70.0	66.7
Vaginal dryness	15.4	10.8	21.5	20.5	19.0	33.3	55.0	61.9
Headaches	24.6	38.6	51.4	42.5	28.6	48.7	50.0	38.1
Depression	27.4	35.0	48.5	50.0	31.0	33.3	37.5	28.6
Mood swings	41.6	31.6	41.6	54.5	50.0	35.9	65.0	45.2
Muscle cramps	2.5	10.0	15.0	15.0	2.4	4.5	5.0	2.4
Acne	21.5	30.0	45.0	51.4	35.7	28.2	22.5	16.7

The most worrying metabolic effect of hypo-oestrogenism is the effect on bone metabolism and induced losses in trabecular bone density. Losses of between 3 and 5% have been detected in trabecular bone density of the lumbar spine following 6 months therapy with GnRH agonists[10,11]. This is reversible, however, in the majority of subjects by 6 months following cessation of treatment[12]. This degree of transient bone density loss over a period of 6 months therapy with GnRH agonists should not be detrimental to eumenorrhoeic women who have normal initial bone mass, but more prolonged courses or repeat courses could have greater consequences unless combined therapies with agents to counteract bone loss are developed.

CONCLUSIONS

GnRH agonists administered over 6 months have proved highly efficacious in achieving endocrine parameters of pituitary desensitization and hypo-oestrogenism. Initial studies treating patients for endometriosis show satisfactory relief of symptoms and significant impact on the disease process as shown by resolution or reduction in number and size of disease deposits. Whether GnRH agonists offer the potential for medical therapy to achieve a long-term resolution of deposits and prevention of recurrence has yet to be evaluated as long-term follow-up studies are undertaken.

ACKNOWLEDGEMENTS

My thanks to Drs Matta, Williams and Gardner who have been Clinical Research Fellows involved in supervising patients with endometriosis in the clinical trials encompassed by this paper.

REFERENCES

1. Meldrum, D.R., Chang, R.J., Lu, J., Vale, W., Rivier, J. and Judd, H.L. (1982). 'Medical oophorectomy' using a long-acting GnRH agonist: a possible new approach to the treatment of endometriosis. *J. Clin. Endocrinol. Metab.*, **54**, 1081–3
2. Shaw, R.W., Fraser, H.M. and Boyle, H. (1983). Intranasal treatment with luteinizing hormone releasing hormone agonist in women with endometriosis. *Br. Med. J.*, **287**, 1667–9
3. Lemay, A., Maheux, R., Faure, N., Jeam, C. and Fazekas, A. (1984). Reversible hypogonadism induced by a luteinizing hormone (LH-RH) agonist (buserelin) as a new therapeutic approach for endometriosis. *Fertil. Steril.*, **41**, 863–71
4. Shaw, R.W. and Matta, W.H. (1986). Reversible pituitary ovarian suppression induced by an LHRH agonist in the treatment of endometriosis: comparison of two dose regimens. *Clin. Reprod. Fertil.*, **4**, 329–36
5. Schriock, E., Monroe, S.E., Henzel, M. and Jaffe, R.B. (1985). Treatment of endometriosis with a potent agonist of gonadotrophin releasing

hormone (nafarelin). *Fertil Steril.*, **44**, 583–8

6. Steingold, K.A., Cedars, M., Lu, J.K.H., Randle, R.N., Judd, H.L. and Meldrum, D.R. (1987). Treatment of endometriosis with a long-acting gonadotrophin releasing hormone agonist. *Obstet. Gynecol.*, **69**, 403–11

7. Matta, W.H. and Shaw, R.W. (1987). A comparative study between buserelin and danazol in the treatment of endometriosis. *Br. J. Clin. Pract.*, **41**, (Suppl. 48), 69–73

8. Henzl, M.R., Corson, S.L., Moghissi, K., Buttram, V.C., Bergqvist, C. and Jacobson, C. (1988). Administration of nasal nafarelin as compared with oral danazol for endometriosis. *N. Eng. J. Med.*, **318**, 485–9

9. Acien, P., Shaw, R.W., Irvine, L., Burford, G. and Gardner, R.L. (1989). CA-125 levels in endometriosis patients before, during and after treatment with danazol or LHRH agonists. *Eur. J. Obstet. Gynecol. & Reprod. Biol.*, **32**, 241–6

10. Matta, W.H., Shaw, R.W., Hesp, R. and Katz, D. (1987). Hypogonadism induced by luteinizing hormone releasing hormone agonist analogue: effects on bone density in premenopausal women. *Br. Med. J.*, **294**, 1523–4

11. Stevenson, J.C., Lees, B., Gardner, R. and Shaw, R.W. (1989). A comparison of the skeletal effects of goserelin and danazol in premenopausal women with endometriosis. *Hormone Research*, **32**, (Suppl. 1), 161–4

12. Matta, W.H., Shaw, R.W., Hesp, R. and Evans, R. (1988). Reversible trabecular bone density loss following induced hypo-oestrogenism with the GnRH analogue buserelin in premenopausal women. *Clin. Endocrinol.*, **29**, 45–51

DISCUSSION

Dr Wheeler

In the very long-term therapy in addition to relative differences between danazol and the agonists on bone, many many epidemiologists are concerned with the effects on the lipids. Would Professor Shaw speculate on that, particularly in reference to his last comment on oestrogen add back?

Prof. Shaw

In terms of 6 month administration courses of a number of analogues there are no significant changes in the lipids that are predictive for arteriosclerotic changes. This is quite the converse with danazol which does have very significant changes, again reversible but maybe of great relevance if repeat or prolonged treatments are used.

Of course, if one starts adding in synthetic oestrogen compounds in addition to the use of agonists, there may be a very different pattern – as seen with oral contraceptives for instance. So we shall have to think carefully about dose, whether this is oestrogen unopposed, or oestrogen plus progestagens. To my knowledge there is no published data as yet on these types of regimes and how that might work.

Prof. Donnez
One of the patients treated with Zoladex continued to menstruate. How can this be explained?

Prof. Shaw
The occurrence of bleeding, spotting episodes in patients taking the analogues, had no correlation with their actual levels of oestrogen. This was perhaps surprising, but not unsurprising if we look at postmenopausal patients who bleed and we find no pathology that have low oestrogens and yet haemorrhages can occur from the endometrium.

There is a general trend of course, that as we lower oestrogens endometrial development is suppressed and menstruation is likely to be inhibited. There must be a threshold in each individual as to when this occurs, or maybe it is an acute change that is necessary to induce bleeding.

Dr Bergqvist
Is the reversal of bone loss after treatment with GnRH as fast and as good if GnRH is given to women aged > 40 who have already started natural bone loss?

Prof. Shaw
All of these women who were being treated for endometriosis, and another cohort as well for whom we have data, were virtually all aged < 40. There is a change in peak bone mass with age and it gradually reduces, and certainly women in their forties are already below their peak bone mass. This is of great concern when we are contemplating using analogue therapy in the perimenopausal patient in that perhaps we may accelerate this process and replacement may not be as effective. This is still to be determined.

8

15

Zoladex in the treatment of pelvic endometriosis: German experiences

K.-W. Schweppe, H. Steinmüller and L. Mettler

INTRODUCTION

Endometriosis is a disease affecting women during their reproductive phase indicating a relationship to the steroid secretion of the ovaries. The most recent attempts in the medical treatment of endometriosis have therefore been based on the suppression of ovarian function. After a phase of stimulation supraphysiological doses of GnRH analogues lead to a reversible down-regulation of the pituitary gland and consequently to suppression of ovarian steroidogenesis. This therapeutic principle has been proven to be effective in the treatment of endometriosis[1] using D-Ser(Bu^t)^6-LHRH(1-9)nonapeptide-ethylamide (buserelin) which has to be applied three times daily intranasally. For several years there has been a GnRH analogue in a depot preparation available – D-Ser-(Bu^t)^6, Azgly^{10} LHRH, Zoladex – which is administered every 4 weeks as a subcutaneous injection[2,3]. In the following paper we report our experiences with this new therapeutic agent for endometriosis.

MATERIAL AND METHODS

In a multicentre study conducted between 1987 and 1989, a total of 102 female patients with laparoscopically and histologicically proven endometriosis were treated with the GnRH agonist goserelin (Zoladex).

In this article we report on the first 74 women where therapy and follow-up period is completed – 52 patients at the Kiel University gynaecological clinic and 22 at the Westerstede gynaecological clinic. The average age was 31 years (range from 20 to 40 years). Endometriosis-induced complaints with or without infertility were reported in 72 women, whereas 30 patients were primarily treated because of infertility alone. Diagnosis of endometriosis was established by laparoscopy and histological examination of biopsies. The degree of disease was assessed by the revised AFS classification. The majority of our patients suffered from endometriosis Stage II (36 women), while 22 belonged to Stage III. Only 12 women were classified as Stage I and another 10 as Stage IV. The GnRH agonist Zoladex was injected subcutaneously as a depot implant each containing 3.6 mg GnRH-A at 4 weekly intervals over a period of 6 months starting on the first day of the menstrual period following diagnostic laparoscopy. On completion of treatment all patients were reassessed at a second-look laparoscopy. Samples for histological examination were taken from persisting endometrial implants and also from obviously healed scar tissue. Before, at monthly intervals during treatment and after an 8 week interval following control laparoscopy, the clinical findings were evaluated: the patients were asked for subjective complaints and side-effects, and venous blood samples were taken for clinical chemistry and hormone assays.

RESULTS

Efficacy of the applied dosage of the GnRH agonist can best be judged on the degree of ovarian suppression as assessed by the serum oestradiol levels (Figure 1). After 4 weeks of therapy, serum oestradiol levels in all patients were below the normal range of the follicular phase. With further usage postmenopausal levels were invariably measured. The progesterone levels were also determined and they clearly showed anovulatory cycles in all patients during the treatment period. Follicle-stimulating hormone (FSH) levels (Figure 2) and LH levels (Figure 3) were slightly suppressed within the normal range; in a few patients the FSH values increased slightly during the course of therapy, probably due to increasing biologically inactive FSH which could not be tested by the radioimmunoassays used. Eight weeks after cessation of therapy, cycle dependent normal values were measured in all patients.

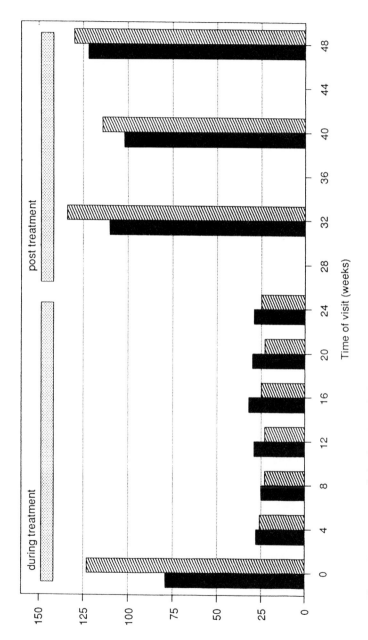

Figure 1 Mean oestradiol values (ng/ml) during and after GnRH analogue treatment with goserelin 3.6 mg monthly.
■ Kiel (*n* = 80); ▨ Westerstede (*n* = 22)

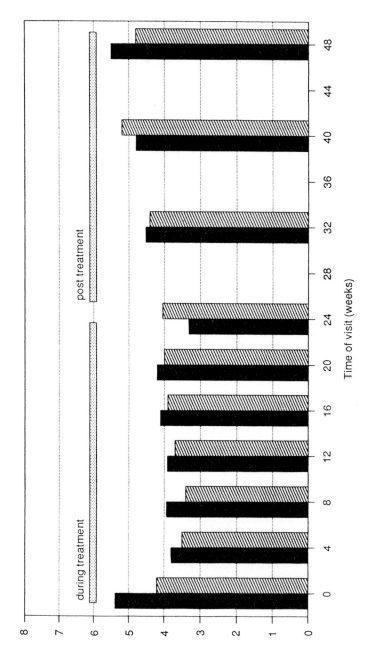

Figure 2 Mean FSH values (mU/ml) during and after GnRH analogue treatment with goserelin 3.6 mg monthly. ■ Kiel (*n* = 80); ▨ Westerstede (*n* = 22)

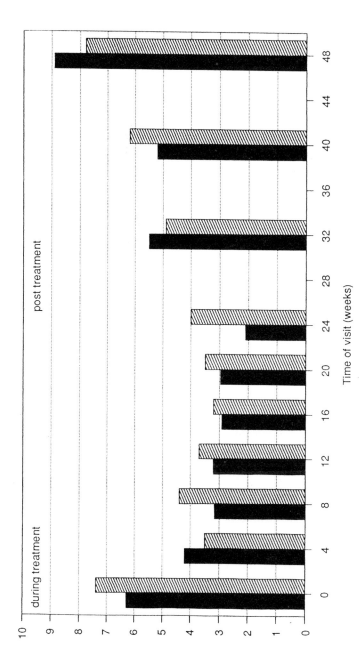

Figure 3 Mean LH values (mU/ml) during and after GnRH analogue treatment with goserelin 3.6 mg monthly. ■ Kiel ($n = 80$); ▨ Westerstede ($n = 22$)

During the treatment period of 6 months the cardinal symptoms, i.e. pelvic pain, dysmenorrhoea and dyspareunia improved in 80–95% of the patients (Figure 4). In the group of patients studied in Kiel the severity of each symptom was judged by a score (0 = absent; 1 = mild; 2 = moderate; 3 = severe) and the total score for each visit is demonstrated in Figure 4. At the end of therapy in both groups 80% of patients were free of pelvic pain and 95% free from dyspareunia. Repeat laparoscopy revealed only 4 patients whose conditions were unchanged and no patient with progression. In all other cases there was a clear regression of at least 50% in the size and number of endometriotic implants. By the criteria of laparoscopic examination in 30 women the endometriosis had disappeared completely (Figure 5).

Fifty-four patients presented with infertility of a mean duration of 3.4 years. Within the follow-up period of 12 months 26 of these had conceived, which represents an uncorrected pregnancy rate in the Kiel group of 47% and in the Westerstede group of 32%. Following conclusion of the treatment, menstrual bleeding first occured within 31 to 66 days after repeat laparoscopy, i.e. 59 to 94 days after the last injection of the depot preparation.

SIDE-EFFECTS

The laboratory parameters examined (white and red blood cell count, clotting parameters, liver enzymes, lipid metabolism, and electrolytes) did not show significant changes, and during and after treatment all values stayed within the normal range of the laboratory. The side-effects of oestrogen deficiency as a result of medical ovarian suppression were the most frequently reported subjective side-effects (Figure 6). In the total group 87% of the patients reported hot flushes – more than 10 times a day – and 70% complained of sweating, especially during the night-time. Decreased libido was observed in 41% and vaginal dryness in 55%. The spectrum of general side-effects was wide and ranged from mild disturbances of well-being to headache, emotional lability and mental depression. Weight gain exceeding 2 kg occurred in isolated cases only. It cannot yet be decided whether these complaints are genuine side-effects of therapy or individual reactions to oestrogen withdrawal. Androgenic side-effects, which are well known from the danazol regimen or from

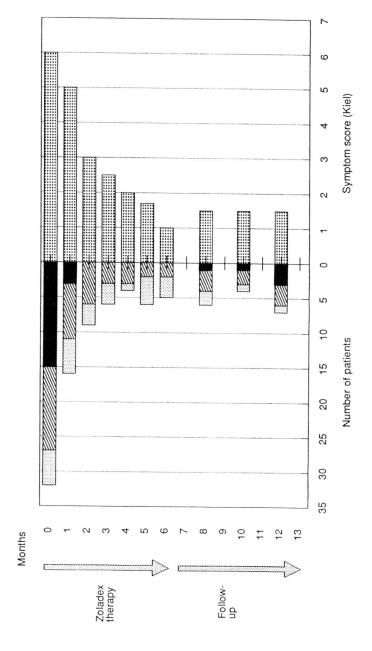

Figure 4 Efficacy of GnRH analogue treatment with goserelin 3.6 mg monthly: subjective complaints during and after therapy. ■ dysmenorrhoea; ▨ pelvic pain; ▨ dyspareunia; ▦ symptoms

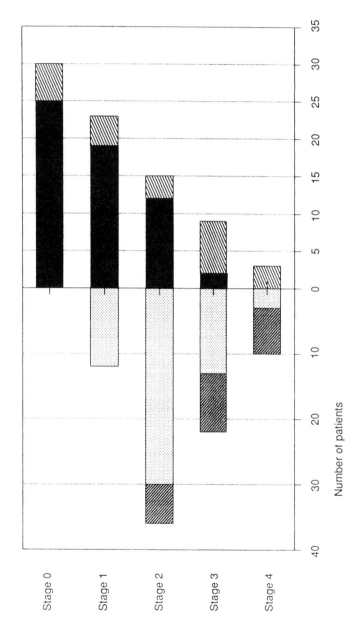

Figure 5 Efficacy of GnRH analogue treatments with goserelin 3.6 mg monthly: score of endometriotic implants. ■ after therapy (Kiel, *n* = 58); ▨ after therapy (Westerstede, *n* = 22); ▦ before therapy (Kiel); ▨ before therapy (Westerstede)

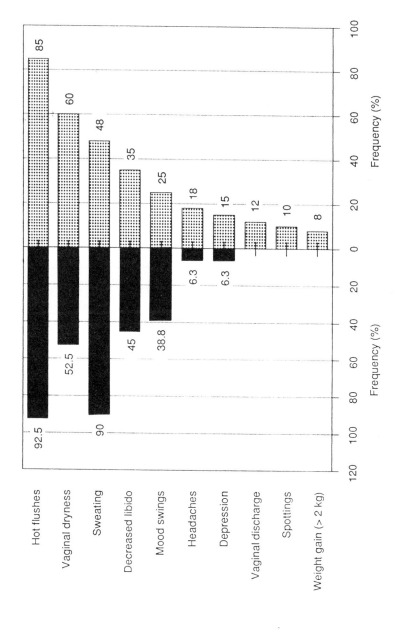

Figure 6 Side-effects during treatment with GnRH analogue goserelin 3.6 mg monthly. ■ Mettler (Kiel); ▦ Schweppe (Westerstede)

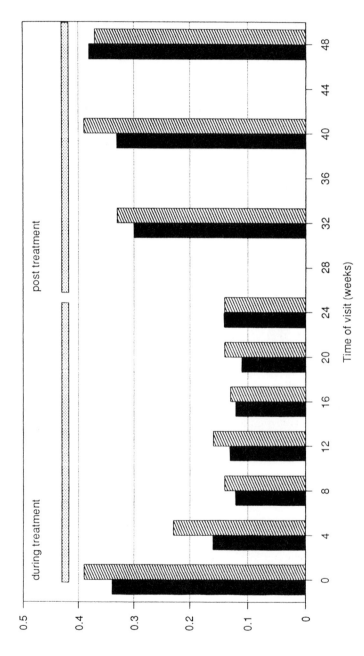

Figure 7 Mean serum testosterone values (ng/ml) during and after therapy with GnRH analogue goserelin 3.6 mg monthly. ■ Kiel (*n* = 80); ▨ Westerstede (*n* = 22)

treatment with gestagens derived from C-19 steroids, were not observed. The total testosterone levels in the serum (Figure 7) showed a significant decrease of more than 50% during treatment and an increase to the pretreatment values 8 weeks after cessation of medication. An unsolved problem, which was not focussed upon in this study, is the risk of osteoporosis during 6 months of medical oophorectomy. Preliminary data using dual photon densiometry and quantitative computed tomography during and after GnRH treatment has demonstrated a significant reduction in the mean lumbar vertebral trabecular bone density of 5.9%, which was reversed within 6 months following resumption of ovarian function[4]. In contrast, there was only a marginal reduction of 0.9% in the mean femoral cortical bone mineral content after 6 months of therapy, which disappeared completely 6 months later[4].

CONCLUSION

Therapy of endometriosis of all stages with the GnRH analogue Zoladex depot in part considerably healed visible endometrial implants and in part caused considerable regression. Complete ovarian suppression was achieved in all patients within 4 weeks. Cyclical ovarian function returned within 2 months of the end of therapy. No unfavourable influences on metabolism were found in this study and subjective side-effects were tolerable and were mainly due to the induced hypo-oestrogenism. The risk of osteoporosis, which may become relevant particularly during long-term therapy, is as yet unclear.

REFERENCES

1. Cirkel, U., Schweppe, K.-W., Ochs, H. and Schneider, H.P.G. (1986). Effects of LH-RH agonist therapy in the treatment of endometriosis (German experiences). In Rolland, R., Chada, D.R. and Willemsen, W.N.P. *Gonadotropin Down-Regulation in Gynecological Practice,* pp. 189–99. (New York: Alan R. Riss)
2. Thomas, E.J., Jenkins, J., Lenton, E.A. and Cooke, I.D. (1986). Endocrine effects of goserelin, a new depot LHRH-agonist. *Br. Med. J.,* **293**, 1407
3. West, C.P., Lumsden, M.A., Lawson, S., Williamson, J. and Baird, D.T. (1987). Shrinkage of uterine fibroids during therapy with goserelin a

LHRH-agonist administered as a monthly s.c. depot. *Fertil. Steril.*, **48**, 45

4. Matta, W.H., Shaw, R.W., Hesp, R. and Evans, R. (1988). Reversible trabecular bone density loss following induced hypoestrogenism with the GnRH analogue buserelin in premenopausal women. *Clin. Endocrinol.*, **29**, 45–51

DISCUSSION

Prof. Shaw
Were there any problems from administering the depot, such as haematomas, any skin reactions or any other problems from the depot itself?

Prof. Schweppe
In Kiel there were no problems and in my group we had no reactions at the site of the injection, but I got one haematoma because I punctured a vessel.

Prof. Donnez
And in our group too there were no skin reactions.

Dr Bayot
Efficacy was judged by excretion of oestradiol. What about the excretion of oestrone, the levels of oestrone in the blood?

Prof. Schweppe
We did not measure oestrone and I have no data.

Dr Bayot
It would be of interest in explaining the differences in reaction to the therapy of the different patients.

Prof. Donnez
The Kiel group reported a 41% pregnant rate. Was this following the hormone therapy alone, or following combined therapy with GnRH agonist and operative laparoscopy?

Prof. Schweppe
The Kiel group performed diagnostic laparoscopy with correction of adhesions at the first laparoscopy but with no additional treatment for the endometriosis. They were then treated, and at repeat laparoscopy they biopsied persistent endometriosis for histological examination, followed by any further surgical treatment.

Prof. Donnez
That is an important observation in respect of the Kiel group's work. It was not true hormonal therapy alone.

16

Zoladex in the treatment of endometriosis : an Italian experience

P.L. Venturini, V. Fasce, S. Costantini, P. Anserini, S. Cucuccio, A. Semino, and L. De Cecco

Although endometriosis is still not completely understood, the finding that women are only affected during their reproductive years strongly supports the concept that ovarian activity is involved in the pathogenesis of endometriosis.

Medical management of endometriosis is directed to interrupt the cyclical changes of oestrogens and progesterone: several compounds, like oral contraceptives, danazol, gestrinone and, more recently, LHRH analogues have been used in pursuit of this aim. LHRH analogues, which produce a down-regulation of the pituitary-ovarian axis, have been proven to induce a reversible medical castration, and this is thought to have beneficial effects on endometriotic implants.

The use of the LHRH analogue buserelin in the management of endometriosis has provided good clinical results, showing both an improvement in symptomatology and a reduction of endometriotic lesions[1-6]. However, a 20–40% incidence of menstrual bleeding, a sign of incomplete suppression of ovarian activity, has been observed[2,5]. The different dosages utilized (300–1200 µg/day intranasally) are the most likely explanation for this finding. However, an inconstant absorption of the drug as a consequence of its mode of administration and the need for repeated injections or nasal insufflations, that sometimes can be missed, should be taken into consideration also. We have also recorded a 25%

incidence of menstrual bleeding with 800 μg/day of buserelin intransasally[7]. In some cases we had to increase temporarily the dose levels of buserelin up to a maximum of 1800 μg/day to avoid further breakthrough bleeding, and this is in accordance with other authors[8].

When Zoladex became available in Italy we decided to test this LHRH analogue for its pharmacokinetic properties and the advantage represented by its monthly administration regimen. This choice has been based on the assumption that a continuous and constant release of the analogue goserelin from its depot could provide a more steady hypothalamic down-regulation and ovarian suppression. At the same time, we were aware that no evidence in the literature supported the real advantage of a complete ovarian suppression in terms of clinical parameters such as pregnancy, pain resolution and incidence of recurrences, as suggested by several studies testing drugs such as danazol, gestrinone or analogues at different dosages[9,10]. The only exception is represented by the paper of the Nafarelin Group[11], in which the authors found a significant improvement in terms of rAFS score only in Stage I patients receiving 800 μg/day in comparision to the 400 μg/day group. This strongly supports the view that during the fertile period of life the degree of ovarian suppression is not the only factor which can condition the history of the disease.

This paper reports our experience with the LHRH analogue goserelin in its depot formulation (Zoladex, ICI).

MATERIALS AND METHODS

Sixty-three patients (mean age ± SD: 28.9 ± 4.1 years) affected by endometriosis diagnosed by laparoscopy or laparotomy were selected for a 6 month period of treatment with Zoladex. The initial depot injections were adminstered in 51 of 63 patients during the early follicular phase, while in the remaining 12 the injections took place in the late luteal phase. Injections were repeated at 28 day intervals for 6 months. Eighteen patients were symptomatic, 25 infertile, and 20 were both symptomatic and infertile. Clinical evaluation (i.e. physical and pelvic examination, evaluation of symptoms of endometriosis and of side-effects) was performed monthly and carried on for a post-treatment follow-up period. Nineteen patients underwent a second-look laparoscopy at the time of the first menstrual bleeding after the end of treatment; this was to assess the efficacy of therapy or eventually carry out conservative surgery at laparotomy when this was indicated. Endocrine effects were evaluated monthly in 32 of 63 patients, 20 of who began the treatment in the early follicular phase of the cycle, while the other 12 began in the late luteal phase. Luteinizing hormone (LH) and follicle-stimulating hormone (FSH) were measured with a monoclonal immunoradiometric assay (IRMA) from Ares-Serono which reacts with the intact molecule so that heterogenous molecules are not detected. Prolactin, 17β-oestradiol(E_2), testosterone, androstenedione, dehydroepiandrosterone sulphate (DHEAS), free testosterone and sex hormone-binding globulin (SHBG) were measured using assays previously described[12].

Statistical analysis was performed using analysis of variance with Bonferroni *t*-test for internal comparison.

RESULTS

Endocrine results

E_2 levels were sharply decreased during treatment with values in the postmenopausal range and a very small standard deviation (Figure 1).

In those who started in the follicular phase, LH serum concentrations were highly significantly decreased ($p < 0.001$) throughout the whole treatment. In the same group FSH was also suppressed, and this suppression was greater and more significant ($p < 0.001$) at the first month: in the subsequent months we observed a gradual increase up to luteal phase levels (fifth and sixth months $p < $ ns). In those who started in the luteal phase, LH and FSH levels show a pattern similar to that observed in the follicular phase starters (Figure 2). Mean values clearly overlap in the two groups of patients during treatment, the difference being only in the initial values. This observation may explain some of the differences reported in the literature about the grade of decrease of gonadotrophins in comparison to the basal levels.

FSH variations under Zoladex therapy seem to be different from those observed with buserelin therapy where, under chronic treatment, the acute administration of large doses elicits a small response in LH and no response in FSH[13]. Lemay and colleagues have showed that after an initial rise of gonadotrophins following subcutaneous buserelin FSH returned to

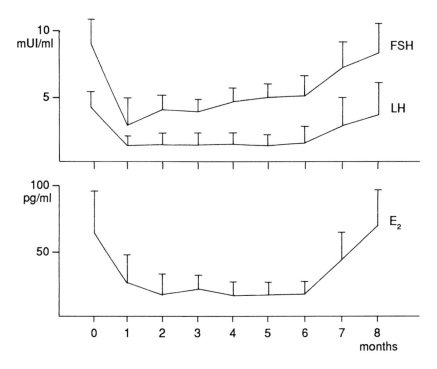

Figure 1 Plasma FSH, LH and 17β-estradiol (E₂) levels (Mean ± SD) before (time = 0), during (1–6) and after therapy with Zoladex every 28 days, administered from time 0 to time 5, in 20 patients starting in the early follicular phase of the cycle

normal levels in 3 days, while LH did so in 2–3 weeks[2]. On the contrary, FSH, and to a lesser degree, LH have been shown to increase following each subsequent implant of Zoladex[14].

Though we do not possess a clear explanation for this effect we do wonder if a lesser suppression of FSH secretion in the presence of very low E₂ levels, and maybe inhibin, might exist. In fact, our monoclonal assay should not react with fractions other than those with biological activity. Although we do not possess experience with higher Zoladex dosages, the data provided by Rittmaster suggest that increasing doses of leuprolide provide only a minimal and not significant decrease of FSH levels[15].

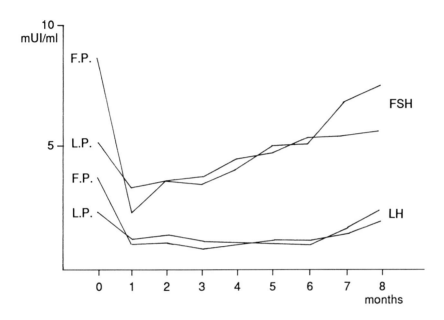

Figure 2 Plasma FSH and LH levels (Mean) before (time = 0), during (1–6) and after therapy with Zoladex every 28 days, administered from time 0 to time 5, in 20 patients starting in the early follicular phase (F.P.) and in 12 starting in the late luteal phase (L.P.) of the cycle

A significant reduction ($p < 0.05$) in total testosterone and a slight, but not significant decrease in androstenedione and SHBG, directly assayed with radioimmunometric kit, were observed during treatment. Conversely, free testosterone, directly assayed, remained practically unchanged (Figure 3). No changes were observed in serum DHEAS concentrations.

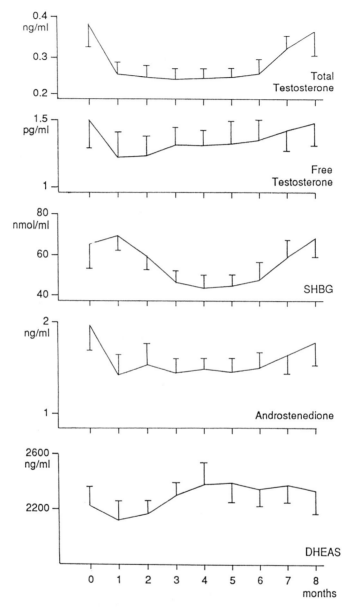

Figure 3 Plasma total testosterone, free testosterone, sex hormone-binding globulin (SHBG), androstenedione and DHEAS levels (Mean ± SEM) before (time = 0), during (1–6) and after therapy with Zoladex every 28 days, administered from time 0 to time 5, in 32 patients

Our data concerning androstenedione are partially in contrast with those produced by West and Baird[16], as we observed that the initial fall was sustained till the end of treatment. It is quite surprising that androstenedione is not significantly decreased. In fact, it has been demonstrated[17-19] that GnRH analogues significantly suppress the ovarian production of androgens in patients with polycystic ovarian syndrome. We ascribe our findings to the possibility that a minimal quantity of gonadotrophins with biological activity may still be present. As a consequence, androstenedione might be produced by those small follicles that we cannot observe at the ultrasound scan. Recently, Williams and colleagues observed that in 8 out of 15 patients with polycystic ovarian syndrome (treated with the GnRH analogue nafarelin) ultrasonography showed neither consistent changes in ovarian size nor the disappearance of ovarian follicles[19]. Data produced by Rittmaster[15] seem to favour a dose–response relationship between analogue and decrease of androgen levels. For this reason we cannot discount the possibility that higher dosages could produce a complete suppression of ovarian androgens. The observation that free testosterone remained unchanged is in accord with the clinical findings. In fact, although typical signs of hypo–oestrogenism are present, we did not observe those of androgenization. SHBG levels remained unchanged in spite of the sharp fall in E_2 levels, probably because of the concomitant reduction of total testosterone levels. Prolactin levels showed a slight decrease without reaching statistical significance.

If we compare the E_2 results from this study with those previously obtained by our group[7] using buserelin 800 μg/day intranasally a more pronounced decrease of E_2 levels can be easily detected in the Zoladex group with a larger standard deviation in the buserelin group (Figure 4). These findings are in agreement with those of Shaw[20] who demonstrated different degrees of E_2 suppression on buserelin, nafarelin, danazol and Zoladex.

Clinical results

All patients became amenorrhoeic after the second injection and no bleeding could be observed in all but one woman who subsequently was diagnosed as having a submucous myoma. The initial bleeding after the

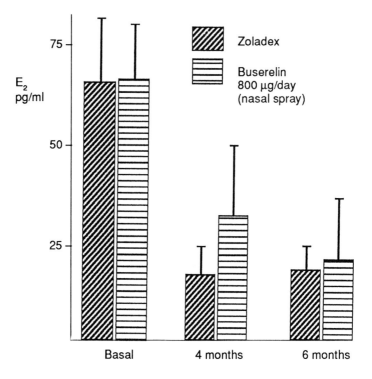

Figure 4 Comparison of plasma 17β-estradiol(E$_2$) levels (Mean ± SD) obtained with Zoladex (32 patients) and buserelin (18 patients). Zoladex data refer to the present study, while buserelin ones have been previously published[7]

first injection was practically identical both in follicular and in luteal phase starters, though in the former bleeding was sometimes longer lasting. Menses returned in all patients 57 – 85 days (mean 67.5) after the last injection. Patients' local tolerance of treatment was very good.

All symptomatic women (38) showed a subjective improvement. Thirty-three complained of mild to severe dysmenorrhoea before treatment (Figure 5). The initial bleeding after the first injection was experienced as moderately painful in 9 out of the 12 patients who began treatment in the late luteal phase and in three of the starters in the follicular phase. During the following months no subsequent complaint of dysmenorrhoea was recorded. Twenty of the 38 patients complained of

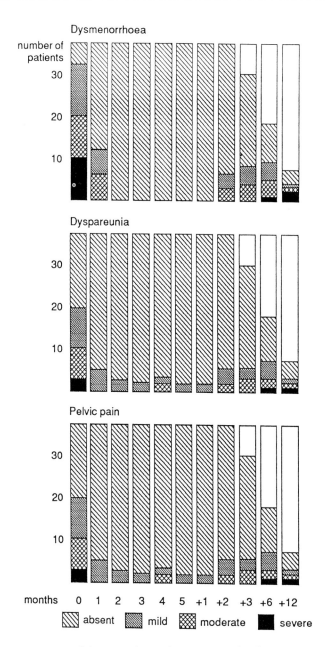

Figure 5 Frequency of dysmenorrhoea, dyspareunia and pelvic pain in 38 patients, during 6 months Zoladex therapy and during follow-up period of 1 year

mild to severe dyspareunia. The frequency of this symptom was sharply decreased during treatment and was always reported as mild or moderate. Half of the patients complained of mild to severe pelvic pain not related to menstruation. At the end of the treatment, pain was still present in one third of these patients but reported as mild or moderate.

Our follow-up observations (6 months) show a recurrence of dysmenorrhoea in 50% of patients (9/18). However, this symptom was improved in all but one patient who still complained of severe dysmenorrhoea. Dyspareunia was reported in 39% (7/18) of patients (one severe, six improved). Pelvic pain was found in 44% (8/18) of patients (none severe, all improved).

Only the completion of the 1 year follow-up for all patients will definitely confirm these preliminary findings. In our study the decrease in symptomatology during treatment and the incidence of recurrences are similar to those obtained with the use of other analogues or other drugs such as gestrinone or danazol[9,10], both on treatment and during the follow-up period.

Regarding side-effects, we have carefully monitored the incidence and the degree of hot flushes, a sign that is thought by some authors to be the leading symptom of an adequate dosage of LHRH analogue. This phenomenon was observed in almost all patients, and we have recorded a small decrease in intensity initially and in incidence later during therapy. The same trend was observed for vaginal dryness, while a decreased libido was noticed in only 28% of patients with its highest incidence at the end of treatment (Figure 6). Patients also complained of cephalea (37%), insomnia (26%), tiredness (25%), mood alterations (21%) and breast discomfort (5%).

The observation that in some patients an increase in blood pressure was found led us to check this sign monthly. We have found a non-significant increase in the systolic values but a widening in the range of their distribution. Diastolic blood pressure levels increased slightly significantly during the first 3 months of treatment. Data are reported in Table 1. In our opinion this phenomenon should be considered not drug dependent but drug related, and it may reflect the change in the reactivity of the neurovascular system like that described in postmenopausal women.

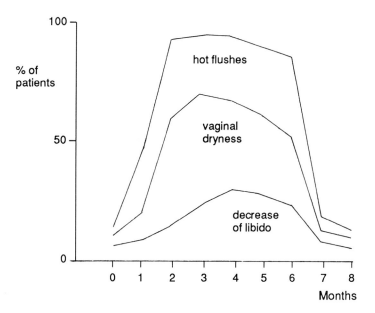

Figure 6 Percentage of incidence of side-effects during 6 months Zoladex therapy

Table 1 Blood pressure evaluation during Zoladex treatment

Month	Diastolic pressure		Systolic pressure	
	Mean	SD	Mean	SD
0	75.1	9.0	119.8	7.9
1	81.8★	13.2	121.6	12.7
2	81.4★	14.1	122.1	12.3
3	78.9★	12.5	125.2	16.6
4	75.2	11.5	117.8	10.8
5	75.2	9.5	115.9	12.4

SD = Standard Deviation
★ = $p < 0.05$ vs basal levels

Laparoscopic findings and pregnancy rates

Nineteen infertile women ($n\,3$ = Stage II; $n\,9$ = Stage III; $n\,7$ = Stage IV) with a mean rAFS score of 29.5 underwent a second laparoscopy after the return of menses. The rAFS scores decreased in all but one patient, reaching a mean of 15.3 (-47.3%). These results are comparable with those reported with danazol, buserelin and nafarelin[5,11]. Adhesions were reduced to a lesser degree (-13.5%).

In the 6 month follow-up group (21 patients) we recorded four pregnancies (pregnancy rate = 27.7%; cumulative pregnancy rate = 0.34). In the 1 year follow-up group (n = 17) two more patients conceived bringing the cumulative rate to 0.42.

CONCLUSIONS

Zoladex, besides having the advantage of its practical depot formulation which ensures a sustained and continuing release of the analogue, provides a very good suppression of gonadal steroidogenesis. E_2 levels during treatment with Zoladex are lower than those found in our experience with 800 μg/day of nasal spray buserelin, although some androgenic activity may still be observed. In fact, although in the literature this therapy is often referred to as 'medical castration', it has been hypothesized that a complete inhibition of gonadal steroidogenesis is rarely achieved with the doses of agonists in current use[21].

Side-effects due to the induced state of hypo-oestrogenism seem to be acceptable. Bone loss observed on treatment with LHRH analogues[22] seems to be reversible at least after a 6 months administration phase.

At this moment we are confident that prolonging the study will not change our endocrine results, but conclusions on the clinical efficacy might be favourably influenced by future data. Our clinical results up to now obtained with Zoladex are comparable with those obtained by other groups with other LHRH analogues or danazol[5,6,11,23].

Finally, we can confirm that the more pronounced inhibition of steroidogenesis obtained with Zoladex does not produce better clinical benefits when compared with other medical treatments. This probably reflects our lack of knowledge as to what level of E_2 can sustain endometriotic tissues along with the fact that there is a reduced presence of E_2 receptors in endometriosis implants[24,25].

REFERENCES

1. Shaw, R.W., Fraser, H.M. and Boyle, H. (1983). Intranasal treatment with luteinizing hormone releasing hormone agonist in women with endometriosis. *Br. J. Obstet. Gynaecol.*, **91**, 913–6

2. Lemay, A., Maheux, R., Faure, N., Jean, C. and Fazekas, A. (1984). Reversible hypogonadism induced by a luteinizing hormone releasing hormone (LH-RH) agonist (buserelin) as a new therapeutic approach for endometriosis. *Fertil. Steril.*, **41**, 863–71

3. Shaw, R.W. and Matta, W. (1986). Reversible pituitary–ovarian suppression induced by an LHRH agonist in the treatment of endometriosis: comparison of two dose regimens. *Clin. Reprod. Fertil.*, **4**, 329–36

4. Matta, W.H. and Shaw, R.W. (1987). A comparative study between buserelin and danazol in the treatment of endometriosis. *Br. J. Clin. Prac.*, **41** (Suppl. 48), 69–73

5. Jelley, R.J. (1986). Multicentre open comparative study of buserelin and danazol in the treatment of endometriosis. *Br. J. Clin. Prac.*, **41** (Suppl. 48), 64–8

6. Lemay, A. (1988). Comparison of GnRH analogues to conventional therapy in endometriosis. *International Symposium on GnRH Analogues*. Geneva, February 18–21, abstract 020

7. Costantini, S., Anserini, P., Valenzano, M., Remorgida, V., Venturini, P.L. and De Cecco, L. (19–). Luteinizing hormone-releasing hormome analog therapy of uterine fibroid: analysis of results obtained with buserelin administred intranasally and goserelin administered subcutaneously as monthly depot. *Eur. J. Obstet. Gynecol. Reprod. Biol.*, (In press)

8. Schweppe, K.W. and Cirkel, U. (1987). GnRH in the treatment of endometriosis. In Teoh, E.S., Ratnam, S.S. and Seng, K.W. (eds.). *Advances in Fertility and Sterility Series*, Vol 5, pp. 27–31. (Carnforth: Parthenon Publishing)

9. Metzger, D.A. and Luciano, A.A. (1989). Hormonal therapy of endometriosis. In Rock, J.A. (ed.). *Obstetrics and Gynecology Clinics of North America*, Vol 16, pp. 105–22. (Philadelphia: W.B. Saunders)

10. Erickson, L.D. and Ory, S.J. (1989). GnRH Analogues in the treatment of endometriosis. In Rock, J.A. (ed.). *Obstetrics and Gynecology Clinics of North America*, Vol 16, pp. 123–45. (Philadelphia: W.B. Saunders)

11. Henzl, M.R., Corson, S.L., Moghissi, K., Buttram, V.C., Berqvist, C. and Jacobson, J. for the Nafarelin Study Group (1988). Administration of nasal nafarelin as compared with oral danazol for endometriosis. A multicenter double-blind comparative clinical trial. *N. Engl. J. Med.*, **318**, 485–9

12. Venturini, P.L., Bertolini, S., Marre Brunenghi, M.C., Daga, A., Fasce, V., Marcenaro, A., Cimato, M. and De Cecco, L. (1989). Endocrine, metabolic, and clinical effects of gestrinone in women with endometriosis. *Fertil. Steril.*, **52**, 589–95

13. Minaguchi, H., Uemura, T. and Shirasu, K. (1986). Clinical study on finding optimal dose of a potent LHRH agonist (buserelin) for the treatment of endometriosis – multicenter trial in Japan. In Rolland, R., Chadha, D.R. and Willemsen, W.N.P. (eds.). *Gonadotrophin Down Regulation in Gynecological Practice,* pp. 211–25. (New York: Alan Liss)

14. Van der Spuy, Z.M., Wood, M., Fieggen, G., Pienaar, C. and Tiltman, A. (1988). GnRH agonist therapy in women with uterine fibroids. Presented at the *International Symposium on Endocrine Therapy.* p. 9. November, Monaco

15. Rittmaster, R.S. (1988). Differential suppression of testosterone and estradiol in hirsute women with the superactive gonadotrophin-releasing hormone agonist leuprolide. *J. Clin. Endocrinol. Metab.*, **67**, 651–5

16. West, C.P. and Baird, D.T. (1987). Suppression of ovarian activity by Zoladex Depot (ICI 118630), a long-acting luteinizing hormone releasing hormone agonist analogue. *Clin. Endocrinol.*, **26**, 213–20

17. Chang, R.J., Laufer, L.R., Meldrum, D.R., De Fazio, J., Lu, J.II., Vale, W.W., Rivier, J.E. and Judd, H.L. (1983). Steroid secretion in polycystic ovarian disease after ovarian suppression by a long-acting gonadotrophin-releasing hormone agonist. *J. Clin. Endocrinol. Metab.*, **56**, 897–903

18. Couzinet, B., Le Strat, N., Brailly, N. and Schaison, G. (1986). Comparative effects of cyproterone acetate or a long-acting gonadotropin-releasing hormone agonist in polycystic ovarian disease. *J. Clin. Endocrinol. Metab.*, **63**, 1031–5

19. Williams, I.A., Shaw, R.W. and Burford, G. (1989). An attempt to alter the pathophysiology of polycystic ovary syndrome using a gonadotrophin hormone releasing hormone agonist – nafarelin. *Clin. Endocrinol.*, **32**, 345–53

20. Shaw, R.W. (1988). LHRH analogues in the treatment of endometriosis – comparative results with other treatments. In Healy, D. (ed.). *Bailliere's Clinical Obstetrics and Gynaecology*, Vol. 2, pp. 659–75

21. West, C.P. (1988). LHRH analogues in the management of uterine fibroids, premenstrual syndrome and breast malignancies. In Healy, D. (ed.). *Bailliere's Clinical Obstetrics and Gynaecology*, Vol. 2, pp. 689–709

22. Matta, W.H., Shaw, R.W., Hesp, R. and Katz, D. (1987). Hypogonadism induced by luteinizing hormone releasing hormone agonist analogues: effects on bone density in premenopausal women. *Br. Med. J.*, **294**, 1523–4

23. Schriock, E., Monroe, S.E., Henzl, M. and Jaffe, R.B. (1985). Treatment of endometriosis with a potent agonist of gonadotrophin releasing hormone (nafarelin). *Fertil. Steril.*, **44**, 583–8

24. Bergqvist, A., Rannevik, G. and Thorell, J. (1981). Estrogen and progesterone cytosol receptor concentration in endometriotic tissue and intrauterine endometrium. *Acta Obst. Gynecol. Scand.*, **101**, 53–8

25. Jänne, O, Kauppila, A., Kokko, E., Lantto, T., Ronnberg, L. and Vihko, R. (1981). Estrogen and progestin receptors in endometriosis lesions: comparison with endometrial tissue. *Am. J. Obstet. Gynecol.*, **141**, 562

DISCUSSION

Prof. Donnez
What is the explanation for the blood pressure variability, because after 6 months of treatment both the mean and the standard deviations of the blood pressure were exactly the same as before treatment.

Prof. Venturini
It is a phenomenon related to neurovascular activity and correlated to the hot flush. It is the same kind of vascular instability that is to be found at menopause in many patients. But it is a problem of the individual patient and not of the group as a whole.

Prof. Donnez
And presumably it could be related to the stress induced by the treatment itself?

Prof. Venturini
Probably.

17

Advances in the surgical management of endometriosis

C. Sutton

INTRODUCTION

Our lack of understanding of the aetiology and pathogenesis of endometriosis is reflected in the plethora of different treatment options available[1]. Against this background it is not surprising, therefore, that both patients and their doctors find themselves confused and frustrated. Before embarking on any management plan it is important to individualize the approach to treatment, because circumstances and situations vary enormously and will depend on the severity of symptoms, previous treatment, the age of the patient and her fertility expectations. If endometriosis is discovered incidentally at the time of laparoscopy it might be perfectly reasonable to advise no treatment at all, especially if the patient is asymptomatic. In the present medico–legal climate, however, it would be prudent to discuss this with the patient because untreated endometriosis may become more severe and give rise to future problems[2].

The rationale behind medical therapy for endometriosis is based on two aspects of the natural history of the disease and on one pharmacological observation: endometriosis usually goes into remission during pregnancy[3,4]; androgens appear to cause regression of the disease[5,6] and endometriosis invariably disappears after the menopause[7]. Drug treatment, therefore, aims to mimic the hormonal state of pregnancy, an androgenic state or the menopause with the inevitable side-effects associated with all these conditions.

Surgical treatment aims to remove the endometriotic implants and can be conservative (if further pregnancies are desired) or radical (with removal of the ovaries to create a menopausal state). Such treatment is usually performed as a last resort when medical therapy has failed.

The most exciting development in endometriosis therapy in recent years has been in the field of laparoscopic surgery, wherein different lasers are used to destroy ectopic endometrial implants. This approach has the overwhelming advantage that effective treatment can be instituted at the same time as the diagnosis is made.

OPERATIVE LAPAROSCOPY

Before the introduction of lasers the only method of removing endometrial implants endoscopically was by relatively crude cutting techniques, or heating the endometrial implants by endocoagulation[8] or destroying them by the passage of an electric current. Uni-polar diathermy can generate high temperatures (up to 600°C) and can damage adjacent tissues such as the ureter or cause serious injury if the bowel is inadvertently touched by the hot instrument[9]. Recently, special laparoscopic surgical instruments (Karl Storz Gmbh, Tuttlingen) have been designed by Hubert Manhes from Vichy, France, and Thierry Vancaille from San Antonio, Texas, and these represent a considerable advance in operative laparoscopy. Although there is certainly a place for removal of implants by laparoscopic scissor excision or diathermy coagulation, the former is rather haemorrhagic and the latter rather imprecise, and in practice it is difficult to be certain that the entire endometrial implant has been removed. The tissue effect of electrodiathermy is such that there is inevitably considerable destruction of surrounding tissue with subsequent fibrosis and scarring, a result that is undesirable in surgery aiming to ensure future fertility. In contrast, the CO_2 laser has the advantage of being able to precisely vaporise abnormal tissue so that, although there is some cellular damage up to 500 μ from the impact point, the zone of thermal necrosis is usually less than 100 μ[10]. Since all the tissue debris is evacuated as smoke in the laser plume there is minimal fibrosis or scar tissue formation and laser wounds heal with virtually no contracture or anatomical distortion[11]. These characteristics make the CO_2 laser particularly suitable for the vaporization of endometriosis and its associated adhesions, especially in patients who are infertile or may wish to have children in the future.

CO_2 LASER LAPAROSCOPY

The first reports of laser laparoscopy came from Clermont-Ferrand in France[12] but prototype instruments and techniques were developed independently in Israel[13], the United States[14], the United Kingdom[15] and Belgium[16].

We started using this technique at St. Luke's Hospital, Guildford in October, 1982 and have treated over 700 patients for a variety of conditions ranging from endometriosis and adhesions to neosalpingo-stomies, ovarian cysts, polycystic ovarian syndrome and unruptured ectopic pregnancies. Hospital stay is relatively short – day case or overnight – and complications are few and usually minor, and we had no injury or morbidity due to laser energy.

CO_2 laser laparoscopy for pelvic pain

We have recently reviewed 228 consecutive patients with endometriosis who were treated by laser laparoscopy between 1982 and 1987 and have been followed up for between 1 and 6 years[17]. Patients were classified according to the presenting symptoms of pain, infertility or both, and all had consented to laser treatment if endometriosis was found at the time of diagnostic laparoscopy. The results are summarized in Figure 1.

Symptomatic improvement was seen in 126 of 181 (70%) of patients complaining of pelvic pain and the benefit was sustained in all but 17 patients who relapsed usually after about 6 months. It is tempting to ascribe this success to the placebo effect of the laparoscopy, but almost a third of these patients had undergone previous laparoscopies or medical therapy without relief of their pain. We managed to persuade 33 patients in this group to have a second-look procedure to evaluate the result of the original laser laparoscopy. In 15 (45.4%) patients there was no evidence of recurrent endometriosis, although the charcoal deposits remaining from the laser vaporization could be clearly seen underneath the peritoneum. Careful inspection with the laparoscope lens held close to the peritoneal

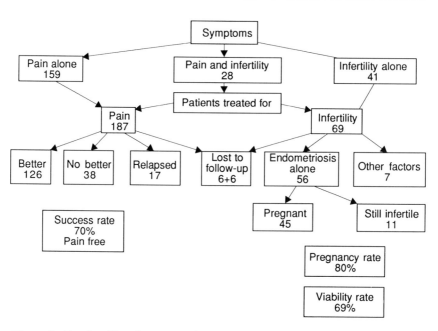

Figure 1   Results of laser laparoscopy in patients with endometriosis (228 patients)

surface revealed a characteristic appearance with no inflammatory reaction, and biopsy showed inactive carbon particles with no evidence of endometrial glands or stroma. The remaining 18 patients (54.6%) had formed endometriosis at different sites but there was no evidence of endometriosis at the sites previously lasered. Obviously this latter group of patients requires medical therapy to prevent further recurrence of the disease.

CO_2 laser laparoscopy for dysmenorrhoea

Many patients with endometriosis suffer from dysmenorrhoea which is usually of the congestive kind, preceding the period by a few days and often partially relieved or changing in character once the bleeding starts. Dysmenorrhoea is particularly likely to be present when there are deposits of endometriosis on or within the uterosacral ligaments. This is almost certainly because the sensory parasympathetic fibres to the cervix and the sensory sympathetic fibres to the corpus traverse the cervical division of the Lee–Frankenhauser plexus which lies in, under and around the attachments of the uterosacral ligaments to the cervix[18]. For many years the operation of presacral neurectomy was employed for patients with intractable dysmenorrhoea, but it yielded disappointing results with failure rates around 11–15% in primary dysmenorrhoea and 25–40% in secondary dysmenorrhoea associated with endometriosis[19–21]. In 1952 White pointed out that the nerve supply to the cervix is not usually interrupted by the presacral neurectomy procedure[22] and then in 1963 Joseph Doyle described the procedure of paracervical uterine denervation that bears his name[23]. The operation was performed abdominally or vaginally, and Doyle pointed out that general surgeons would prefer the former approach whereas gynaecologists would be more comfortable with a vaginal procedure. The results were extremely impressive with complete pain relief in 63 out of 73 cases (86%), and the results were equally good for primary or secondary dysmenorrhoea. With such a satisfactory outcome it is difficult to see why this relatively simple procedure has been condemned to oblivion. Possibly the development of potent non-steroidal anti-inflammatory drugs (NSAIDs) and ovulation suppressants has reduced the demand for relatively drastic surgical intervention. Interest in Doyle's work has recently revived with the development of surgical lasers which can be used endoscopically and which will perform much the same tissue effect without the need for major surgery[24–26].

During the past 5 years we have treated 126 patients with laser uterine nerve ablation (LUNA) laparoscopically[26]. Of the group of patients, 26 had primary dysmenorrhoea and 100 had secondary dysmenorrhoea associated with endometriosis. We did not include patients with secondary dysmenorrhoea due to other causes such as fibroids, adenomyosis or pelvic congestion.

In the endometriosis group six patients were lost to follow-up but 81 (86%) reported an improvement in symptoms, even though 26 (32%) of them had a partial (unilateral) neurectomy. In three patients the symptoms returned at 6 months to 1 year following the procedure. No patients were made worse, but 13 reported no improvement and, interestingly, nine of these had incomplete or partial neurectomies due to poor formation of the ligaments resulting in difficulty in localizing and vaporizing the nerve bundles.

There were no serious complications in this group of patients and all were treated on a day case or overnight stay basis. Troublesome bleeding was encountered in two patients, requiring endocoagulation or haemostatic clips and the insertion of a redivac drain for the pelvis for several hours postoperatively.

Feste has recently reported on a larger series from Houston[27]. He performed laser neurectomy on 196 patients with intractable dysmenorrhoea who had failed to respond to traditional therapy. Of the 124 patients that he managed to follow up the failure rate was only 12.9%, which is almost exactly the same result as that obtained by us.

Both the above series suffer from the disadvantage that they are entirely retrospective and uncontrolled, and sceptics can quite reasonably argue that there is a massive placebo effect with this kind of symptom and this kind of high-tech surgery. The study of Lichten and Bombard is therefore particularly interesting because it is one of the few, or indeed the only, randomized prospective double-blind study in the entire field of operative laproscopy. A relatively homogeneous group of women was selected who had severe or incapacitating dysmenorrhoea, who had no demonstrable pelvic pathology at laparoscopy and who were unresponsive to NSAIDs and oral contraceptives prescribed concurrently. Coexisting psychiatric illness was evaluated with the Minnesota Multiphasic Personality Inventory, and those with an abnormal psychological profile were excluded from the study. The remaining 21 patients were randomized to uterine nerve ablation or control group at the time of the diagnostic laparoscopy. Neither the patient nor the clinical psychologist who conducted the interview at the follow-up were aware of the group to which the patient had been randomized. No patient in the control group reported relief from dysmenorrhoea, whereas 9 of the 11 patients (81%) who had LUNA reported almost complete relief at 3 months and five of them had continued relief from dysmenorrhoea 1 year after surgery. Interestingly those that reported surgical success also reported relief from the associated symptoms of nausea, vomiting, diarrhoea and headaches[28]

CO_2 laser laparoscopy and dyspareunia

Patients with endometriosis complaining of deep dyspareunia are usually found to have active telangiectatic or vesicular implants in the cul-de-sac or deposits in the uterosacral ligaments which are responsible for the nodular feeling when such patients are examined vaginally. When using the CO_2 laser to eradicate these nodules it is important to continue vaporization at a relatively high power density until no futher haemosiderin is released and until the assistant confirms that no further nodules are palpable on vaginal and rectal examination.

Sometimes adhesions are present between the rectum and the posterior aspect of the cervix, and this is often responsible for the dyspareunia. In its extreme form this eventually develops into partial or complete obliteration of the cul-de-sac, giving rise to a high score on the AFS scale. Paradoxically, however, many patients with complete obliteration of the cul-de-sac do not mention dyspareunia among their symptoms, whereas some patients with a few active deposits are acutely uncomfortable during deep penetrations and the discomfort continues as a nagging ache well into the following day.

It is important to rid the cul-de-sac of all adhesions and implants in order to alleviate discomfort during intercourse. Care must be taken when using the laser over the rectum itself and the power-density should be reduced and, until considerable experience has been amassed, the laser should be used on a pulsed mode with repeated irrigation to remove the charcoal and assess the depth of destruction in relation to the anatomy of the rectal wall. With experience the beam can be used on continuous mode with rapid hand movement to prevent penetration of the rectal mucosa. In patients with complete obliteration of the cul-de-sac it is necessary to use the laser to open up a plane of cleavage between the cervix and the rectum and to use aqua-dissection to extend this. These techniques of advanced operative laparoscopy have been pioneered by Reich from Kingston, Pennsylvania, and most of his early results were achieved with conventional operative laparoscopy and only in recent years has he been converted to the use of the CO_2 laser[29].

In our retrospective study we did not specifically enquire about dyspareunia in our analysis of the results, although our impression is that most patients with active disease in the posterior fornix have benefitted from laser treatment. Donnez reported on a series of 100 patients who have been followed for more than a year after LUNA. He found that most patients complaining of dyspareunia experienced relief from this symptom following the operation. We have noticed that even in the absence of visible endometriosis patients with very taut uterosacral ligaments seem to complain of dyspareunia which is relieved by the simple act of dividing the ligaments with the laser. This may be a purely physical effect or it could be due to the fact that in 52% of patients with infertility but no macroscopic evidence of endometriosis biopsies from the uterosacral ligaments reveal endometrial glands and stroma on histological examination[30].

CO_2 laser laparoscopy for infertility

Although there is little doubt that gross anatomical distortion caused by severe endometriosis is reponsible for infertility, some authors have suggested that the relationship with early stage disease is incidental rather than causal[31].

In the Guilford series there were 56 patients with endometriosis as the only abnormal factor implicated in their infertility, which had ranged from 6 months to 10 years. Of these patients 45 (80%) have become pregnant following laser laparoscopy, without adjuvant drug treatment – the majority (73%) within 8 months of the procedure[26].

Our data compare favourably with results from the United States[32–35,27] and Europe[16]. In 1986 Nezhat obtained 62 pregnancies in 102 patients which included one elective termination and nine spontaneous abortions. Our abortion rate was even higher (26%) which probably reflects the high abortion rate noted among endometriosis sufferers[36]. If the results are presented as the 'take home' baby rate our viability rate was 69%. The results of several recent studies are published in Table 1. They can all be criticized on the basis that they are retrospective studies, and there is a great need for a double-blind randomized prospective study comparing laser treatment with expectant management. Such a trial is under way at the present time in our hospital but, with the benefit of hindsight, we wish we had started it 7 years ago before we had established a reputation for laser laparoscopic surgery. We are now finding it almost impossible to recruit new patients into the study who know that they may get no treatment at all.

ARGON AND KTP/532 LASER LAPAROSCOPY

The main advantage of the CO_2 laser is precision but, at the present time, commercially available lasers of this type can only be passed down rigid

Table 1 Results of laser laparoscopy for endometriosis

Authors	Patients	Pregnancies		Viability
	n	n	%	%
Daniell[32]	40	20	50	–
Feste[24]	29	21	72	–
Davis[34]	65	37	–	57
Nezhat[33]	102	62	61	51
Donnez[16]	70	40	–	57
Sutton*[17]	56	45	80	69
Feste*[27]	64	52	81	–

* Endometriosis alone, no other infertility factors

delivery systems with multiple mirrors. This tends to be rather cumbersome, can cause loss of beam alignment and can be difficult to use in places where access is difficult – such as the posterior surface of an ovary that is adherent to the broad ligament. The neodymium-YAG, the argon and the KTP/532 lasers can all be passed down flexible fibres and have the added advantage that they will work in haemorrhagic fields, whereas CO_2 laser energy is absorbed by blood rendering it ineffective. The physical properties of these lasers is summarized in Table 2.

As can be seen, the argon and the potassium-titanyl-phosphate laser (KTP/532, a frequency-doubled YAG laser) are of virtually the same wavelength and are in the blue-green portion of the spectrum, and as such there is selective absorption of energy by haemoglobin and haemosiderin, both of which are present in abundant amounts within the endometrial implants. It is a myth, however, to think that this laser–tissue interaction prevents damage to surrounding structures. In fact, the primary tissue reaction is coagulation with lateral thermal damage of 0.5 – 2 mm, less than with the neodymium-YAG but much more than that produced by the CO_2 laser. In addition, at higher energy levels when tissue vaporizes and carbon builds up, further attempts at lasering through this will result in incandescence as tissue heats with an orange glow to over 1500°. This could cause extensive thermal damage resulting in a branding-iron type of burn and ultimate scarring of tissue[37]. In view of these problems and the

Table 2 Properties of surgical lasers

	CO_2	Nd:YAG	Argon	KTP/532
Wavelength	10.6 μm	1.06 μm	0.5 μm	0.532 μm
Primary tissue effect	Vaporization	Coagulation	— Coagulation —	
Colour dependent	No	Yes	Yes	Yes
Effect on water	Strongly absorbed	Slightly absorbed	Not absorbed	Not absorbed
Scattering of beam	None	Moderate	Slight	Slight
Fibre transmission	No	Yes	Yes	Yes
Depth of tissue effect	0.1 mm	4 mm	1–2 mm	1–2 mm

eye hazards inherent in their use these lasers should only be used by laparoscopists already adept at CO_2 laser laparoscopy.

The first animal and human studies with the argon laser used laparoscopically were performed by Professor William Keye at the University of Utah and with the KTP/532 laser by Jim Daniell in Nashville, Tennessee. Keye reported a prospective study involving 92 consecutive patients who were evaluated for ability to conceive and reduction of pain. Many of the patients had additional sub-fertility factors and 34% became pregnant (a monthly fecundity rate of 2.5%) and 64% of these were within 6 months of treatment. More dramatic was the relief of pain in 92% of 50 women who were complaining of dyspareunia, dysmenorrhoea and pelvic pain due to endometriosis[38].

Using the KTP/532 laser combined with LUNA (laser uterine nerve ablation) Daniell achieved a 75% relief of dysmenorrhoea in endometriosis patients[39]. Nezhat compared the CO_2, argon and KTP/532 lasers in three groups of 40 patients and found the best outcome in terms of pain relief and pregnancy with the CO_2 laser[40].

NEODYMIUM-YAG LASER LAPAROSCOPY

This is a solid state laser in which the crystal of yttrium aluminium garnet is deliberately contaminated with neodymium ions which then becomes the actual lasing medium. It can be passed down flexible fibres, it works in a liquid medium and it generates less smoke than the CO_2 laser. It is absorbed by all tissues to a depth of 3–5 mm and is therefore excellent for haemostasis. Unfortunately, however, there is up to 40% of back-scatter which at this wavelength could damage permanently the macula portion of the retina and lead to blindness; as a consequence, special goggles have to be worn by all theatre personnel.

Lomano first reported its use on 60 cases of early endometriosis with acceptable results[41], and Corson has recently reported on 100 patients, 60 of whom had Stages III and IV disease, many of whom had failed to respond to medical or surgical treatment. Conception occurred for 41% within 9 months, and 63% had complete pain relief with partial relief in a further 29%[42].

In Guildford we have used the neodymium-YAG laser for the past 2 years. It has the slight disadvantage that the equipment takes more time to set up and requires more stringent safety precautions than does the CO_2 laser and this can be a problem during a busy surgical schedule. The problem of beam scatter and the laser–tissue interaction means that it is less precise but this can be partially overcome by the use of artificial sapphire laser scalpels. These are particularly useful in situations where bleeding can be expected, but they have a limited life span, are expensive and tend to stick to tissues if not used correctly. All fibre lasers generate less smoke and are particularly useful in laparoscopic ovarian surgery.

LASER LAPAROSCOPY FOR OVARIAN ENDOMETRIOMAS

Ovarian endometriomas (chocolate cysts) are notorious for their poor response to danazol and progestagens. They can be removed laparoscopically by scissors and blunt dissection but the procedure is time consuming, difficult and at the same time relatively crude. A more sophisticated approach is to make a linear incision over the thinnest part of the endometrioma capsule with argon, KTP/532 or neodymium-YAG laser at a power setting of 10–15 watts. The old blood and haemosiderin (chocolate fluid) inside the cyst is sucked out and the cavity repeatedly irrigated with heparinised Hartmann's solution. The laser fibre is then introduced inside the cyst to photocoagulate the cyst wall at 5–10 watts.

There is no need for the insertion of endosutures, and the cyst can be left open to heal over.

An interesting new technique for dealing with ovarian endometriomas has recently been described by Brosens. For ovarian cystoscopy (ovarioscopy) he uses a double optic laparoscope which is a combination of an operating laparoscope and a 2.6 mm rigid endoscope inside a 5 mm sheath which is introduced down the operating channel of the laparoscope. The sheath is necessary to provide a 1 mm channel for the passage of biopsy forceps, laser fibres and irrigating solutions.

The cyst is punctured and the contents aspirated and sent for cytological examination. The ovarioscope is then introduced through the puncture hole and the cyst distended with continuous flow of saline until the solution becomes clear so that the inner wall can be inspected and biopsied. Once the operator is satisfied that this is a benign ovarian cyst, an argon laser fibre is introduced to photocoagulate the superficial vessels and haemorrhagic areas lining the cyst wall to a depth of 1–2 mm. In a 6 month follow up of 11 patients treated by this technique there have been no recurrences of ovarian endometriomas[43].

CONSERVATIVE SURGERY

This type of surgery is usually reserved for patients with moderate or severe disease who wish to retain or improve their fertility prospects. The rationale behind this approach must be seriously questioned because the only two studies providing monthly fecundity rates demonstrate a similar rate of conception to those treated with danazol or even expectant management[44,45]. Microsurgical techniques should be employed wherever possible and this implies gentle tissue handling, meticulous haemostasis, the use of some form of magnification and constant irrigation to prevent dessication of tissues and subsequent adhesion formation. There is possibly still an indication for this type of surgery for removal of ovarian endometriomata or for performing uterine ventrosuspension, but both of these procedures can be performed more simply by laparoscopy with less risk of adhesion formation and less morbidity. Presacral neurectomy can relieve central pelvic pain and dysmenorrhoea in up to 75% of patients[20], but this can be achieved much more simply by laser uterine nerve ablation (vaporization of the uterosacral ligaments) performed laparoscopically[39].

Lasers have been used at laparotomy via an operating microscope[46] but the results were not significantly better than those obtained by laser laparoscopy or even over conventional operative laparoscopy[47].

CONCLUSION

The scientific study of the treatment of endometriosis has suffered from the large number of poorly designed and uncontrolled trials which makes it difficult to provide clearly defined guidelines for the management of our patients. Several double-blind randomized prospective studies are now under way, but it will be several years before these provide meaningful data.

At this moment in time it appears that it is advantageous to treat the visible endometriotic implants with laser vaporization at the same time as the laparoscopic diagnosis is made. The monthly fecundity rate is high, regardless of the stage of the disease, and the patient avoids having to delay conception.

If laser equipment is not available then endocoagulators or bipolar diathermy are a possible alternative, as long as caution is exercised in the vicinity of bowel, bladder and ureter.

If patients relapse or fail to get pregnant after a year, consideration should be given to drug therapy or assisted conception techniques. If pain is the dominant symptom and laparoscopic or conservative surgery fails, then danazol or LHRH analogues are often effective for short-term therapy and progestagens are suitable for long-term suppression. The final eradication of the disease awaits the menopause either naturally or surgically, but if the latter is employed it is essential to remove all ovarian tissue, and in the presence of dense endometriotic adhesions and the proximity of the ureter this is not always easy to achieve.

This fascinating and perplexing disease has suffered from a surfeit of anecdotal data gleaned from retrospective and uncontrolled trials against a natural background pregnancy rate, which is further complicated by difficulties in sorting out the physical and psychological elements associated with the perception of pelvic pain. There is an urgent need for randomized prospective controlled studies to help us determine the best treatment options available to our patients.

REFERENCES

1. Sutton, C.J.G. (1990). The treatment of endometriosis. In Studd, J.W.W. (ed.). *Progress in Obstetrics and Gynecology.* Vol. 8 (London: Churchill Livingstone) (In press)
2. Thomas, E.J. and Cooke, I.D. (1987). Successful treatment of endometriosis: does it benefit infertile women? *Br. Med. J.,* **294**, 1117–9
3. Meigs, J.V. (1938). Endometriosis, a possible aetiological factor. *Surgery, Gynaecol. and Obstet.,* **67**, 253
4. Kistner, R.W. (1959). The treatment of endometriosis in inducing pseudopregnancy with ovarian hormones: a report of 58 cases. *Fertil. Steril.,* **10**, 539
5. Hamblen, E.C. (1957). Androgen treatment of women. *South. Med. J.,* **50**, 743
6. Greenblatt, R.B. and Tzingounis, V. (1979). Danazol treatment of endometriosis: long term follow-up. *Fertil. Steril.,* **32**, 518
7. Shaw, R.W. (1988). LHRH analogues in the treatment of endometriosis – comparative results with other treatments. In Healy, D. (ed.). *Anti-hormones in Clinical Gynaecology.* vol 2, **3**
8. Semm, K. and Mettler, L. (1980). Technical progress in pelvic surgery via operative laparoscopy. *Am. J. Obstet. Gynecol.,* **138**, 121–7
9. Chamberlain, G.V.P. (1982). *Gynaecological Laparoscopy. The Report of the Working Party of the Confidential Enquiry into Gynaecolgical Laparoscopy.* (London: Royal College of Obstetricians and Gynaecologists)
10. Bellina, J.H., Hemmings, R., Voros, I.J. and Ross, L.F. (1984). Carbon dioxide laser and electrosurgical wound study with animal model. A comparison of tissue damage and healing patterns in peritoneal tissue. *Am. J. Obstet. Gynecol.,* **148**, 327
11. Allen, J.M., Stein, D.S. and Shingleton, H.M. (1983). Regeneration of cervical epithelium after laser vaporization. *Obstet. Gynecol.,* **62**, 700–4
12. Bruhat, M.A., Mage, C. and Manhes, H. (1979). Use of CO_2 laser via laparoscopy. In Kaplan, I. (ed.). *Laser Surgery III. Proceedings of the 3rd Congress of the International Laser Society.* pp. 275. (Tel Aviv: International Society for Laser Surgery)
13. Tadir, Y., Kaplan, I. and Zuckerman, Z. (1981). A second puncture probe for laser laparoscopy. In Atsumi, K. and Nimsakul, N. (eds.). *Laser Surgery IV. Proceedings of the Fourth Congress of the International Society for Laser Surgery.* pp. 25–26. (Tokyo: International Society for Laser Surgery)
14. Daniell, J.F. and Brown, D.H. (1982). Carbon dioxide laser laparoscopy: initial experience in experimental animals and humans. *Obstet. Gynecol.,* **59**, 761

15. Sutton, C.J.G. (1986). Initial experience with carbon dioxide laser laparoscopy. *Lasers in Med. Sci.*, **1** 25–31

16. Donnez, J. (1987). CO_2 laser laparoscopy in infertile women with endometriosis and women with adnexal adhesions. *Fertil. Steril.*, **48**, 390–4

17. Sutton, C.J.G. and Hill, D. (19—). Laser laparoscopy in the treatment of endometriosis. A five year study. *Br. J. Obstet. Gynaecol.* (In press.)

18. Campbell, R.M. (1950). Anatomy and histology of sacro-uterine ligaments. *Am. J. Obstet. Gynecol.*, **59**, 1–7

19. Tucker, A.W. (1947). Evaluation of pre-sacral neurectomy in the treatment of dysmenorrhoea, *Am. J. Obstet. Gynecol.*, **53**, 226

20. Ingersoll, F. and Meigs, J.V. (1948). Presacral neurectomy for dysmenorrhoea. *N. Engl. J. Med.*, **238**, 340–57

21. Polan, M.L. and DeCherney, A. (1980). Presacral neurectomy for pelvic pain in infertility. *Fertil. Steril.*, **34**, 557–9

22. White, J.C. (1952). Conduction of visceral pain. *N. Engl. J. Med.*, **246**, 686

23. Doyle, J.B. and Des Rosiers, J.J. (1963). Paracervical uterine denervation for relief of pelvic pain. *Clin. Obstet. Gynec.*, **6**, 742–53

24. Daniell, J.F. (1985). Laser laparoscopy. In Keye, W.R. (ed.). *Laser Surgery in Obstetrics and Gynaecology,* pp. 147–63. (Boston: G.K. Hall)

25. Feste, J.R. (1985). Laser laparoscopy: a new modality. *J. Reprod. Med.*, **30**, 413–8

26. Sutton, C.J.G. (1989). Laser laparoscopic uterine nerve ablation. In Donnez, J. (ed.). *Operative Laser Laparoscopy and Hysteroscopy,* pp. 43–52. (Louvain, Belgium: Nauwelaerts Publishers)

27. Feste, J.R. (1989). Personal communication

28. Lichten, E.M. and Bombard, J. (1987). Surgical treatment of primary dysmenorrhoea with laparoscopic uterine nerve ablation. *J. Reprod. Med. J.*, **295**, 6591

29. Reich, H. (1989). Advanced operative laparoscopy. In Sutton, C.J.G. (ed.). *Laparoscopic Surgery.* pp. 655–81. (London: Bailliere Tindall)

30. Nisolle, M., Paindareine, B., Bourdon, A., Casanas, F. and Donnez, J. (1989). Peritoneal endometriosis: typical aspects and subtle appearances. In Donnez, J. (ed.). *Operative Laser Laparoscopy and Hysteroscopy,* pp. 25–41. (Louvain, Belgium: Nauwelaerts Publishers)

31. Lilford, R.J. and Dalton, M.E. (1987). Effectiveness of treatment for infertility. *Br. Med. J.*, **295**, 6591

32. Daniell, J.F. (1985). Operative laparoscopy for endometriosis. *Seminars in Reprod. Endocrinol.*, **3**, 353–9

33. Nezhat, C., Crowgey, S.R. and Garrison, C.P. (1986). Surgical treatment of endometriosis via laser laparoscopy. *Fertil. Steril.*, **45**, 778–83

34. Davis, G.D. (1986). Management of endometriosis and its associated

adhesions with the carbon dioxide laser laparoscope. *Obstet. Gynecol.*, **68**, 422–5

35. Nezhat, C., Winer, W., Crowgey, S. and Nezhat, F. (1989). Videolaseroscopy for endometriosis. *Fertil. Steril.*, **51**, 237–40

36. Malinak, L.R. and Wheeler, J.M. (1985). Association of endometriosis with spontaneous abortion; prognosis for pregnancy and risk of recurrence. *Seminars in Reproductive Endocrinology*, **3**, 361–9

37. Absten, G. (1990). Physics of light and lasers. In Sutton, C.J.G. (ed.). *Lasers in Gynaecology* (London: Chapman and Hall) (In press)

38. Keye, W.R. and Dixon, J. (1983). Photocoagulation of endometriosis by the argon laser through the laparoscope. *Obstet. Gynecol.*, **62**, 383–6

39. Daniell, J.F. (1990). Advanced operative laser laparoscopy. In Sutton, C.J.G. (ed.). *Lasers in Gynaecology* (London: Chapman and Hall) (In press)

40. Nezhat, C., Winer, W. and Nezhat, F. (1988). A comparison of the carbon dioxide, Argon and KTP/532 lasers in the videolaseroscopic treatment of endometriosis. *Colposcopy and Gynecol. Laser Surgery.*, **4**, 41–7

41. Lomano, J.M. (1985). Photocoagulation of early pelvic endometriosis with the neodymium-YAG laser through the laparoscope. *J. Reprod. Med.*, **30**, 77–9

42. Corson, S.L. (1990). Laparoscopic applications of the neodymium-YAG laser. In Sutton, C.J.G. (ed.). *Lasers in Gynaecology* (London: Chapman and Hall) (In press)

43. Brosens, I.A. and Puttemans, P.J. (1989). Double optic laparoscopy. In Sutton, C.J.G. (ed.). *Laparoscopic Surgery. Baillières Clinical Obstetrics and Gynaecology* vol. 3, **3**, 595–608.

44. Guzick, D.S. and Rock, J.A. (1983). A comparison of danazol and conservative surgery for the treatment of infertility due to mild or moderate endometriosis. *Fertil. Steril.*, **40**, 580–3

45. Olive, D.L. and Lee, K.L. (1986). Analysis of sequential treatment protocols for endometriosis associated infertility. *Am. J. Obstet. Gynecol.*, **154**, 613–16

46. Chong, A.P. and Baggish, M.S. (1984). Management of pelvic endometriosis by means of intra-abdominal carbon dioxide laser. *Fertil. Steril.*, **41**, 14–19

47. Reich, H. and McGlynn, F. (1986). Treatment of ovarian endometriomas using laparoscopic surgical techniques. *J. Reprod. Med.*, **31**, 577–84

DISCUSSION

Dr Cornillie
What is Mr Sutton's surgical approach to peritoneal pouches? What does he really do with them?

Mr Sutton
There are two approaches. One is to open up a plane of cleavage with the laser and then use aqua dissection to try and break down all the adhesions, and then try to vaporize as much of the endometriosis as we can. The other technique is to use the laser to excise the tissue, which has the advantage that it can be sent for biopsy. Both techniques have good results.

Dr Malinak
Is there data on second-look laparoscopy in patients in whom laparoscopic vaporization of the uterosacral ligaments was performed?

Mr Sutton
For a few. We cannot in all honesty with such good results find very many who need to have a second look.

Dr Malinak
What about adhesions of the Fallopian tubes and ovaries to those sites?

Mr Sutton
We have seen none at all, but I have only had two that I have had a second look at. Both of those had adenomyosis and I had a second look at hysterectomy. In those two the uterosacrals had healed right over, which one would expect, but there was no adhesion formation at all.

Prof Donnez
I have a similar comment. Following ablation with the laser at second-look laparoscopy only a very few showed adhesions. It is very rare.

It was suggested that there is no need to use drugs for laser surgery. But there is probably another concept. I use combined therapy for the very large cysts and one of the advantages of pre-operative hormonal therapy in cases of very large endometrioma, > 3–4 cm, is that it reduces ovarian size and facilitates surgery by laser laparoscopy.

Mr Sutton

I am really not convinced that it works. I have had several patients who I have delayed operating on recently because they have had big ovarian endometriomas. We put them on LHRH analogues and they have come back all of them with cysts that have been bigger. So I am just not convinced that it really works.

Prof Donnez

I do not get exactly those results. The technique I use for the very large endometrioma is not total excision. I vaporize the wall of the ovarian cyst and this technique can be facilitated by using pre-operative GnRH agonists because the epithelium, the lining of the ovarian cyst, is then less inflammatory. In my own series the size of the cyst is reduced in most cases by 25–30%.

Dr Cornillie

For the treatment of ovarian endometriotic cyst a new technique that was proposed by Professor Brosens may be in some ways misleading. I have looked at the cyst wall by histopathology in several cases and quite frequently I have seen secondary small cyst formation in the wall. These secondary small cysts can measure 1–2 mm in the wall of a large cyst and they are deep enough and cannot be eradicated just by lasering the internal surface of the cyst wall. And so if this is left there may be a problem of subsequent recurrence and it may be better to excise the whole wall and to dissect it free.

Index